HORMONE LIES
And Thyroid Misunderstandings

A Medical Intuitive Reveals the Truth
Behind the World's Hormone and Thyroid Crisis

Dr. Emil Faithe

Edited by Dick Brown

Published by BookLocker.com, Inc., Bradenton, Florida.

Printed in the United States of America.

BookLocker.com, Inc.
2013

First Edition

Disclaimer

The author, editor, and publisher are providing this book and its contents on an "as is" basis and make no representations or warranties of any kind with respect to this book or its contents. The author, editor, and publisher disclaim all such representations and warranties, including for example warranties of merchantability and healthcare for a particular purpose. In addition, the author, editor, and publisher do not represent or warrant that the information accessible via this book is accurate, complete or current.

The statements made about products and services have not been evaluated by the U.S. Food and Drug Administration. They are not intended to diagnose, treat, cure, or prevent any condition or disease.

Except as specifically stated in this book, neither the author, editor, or publisher, nor any authors, contributors, or other representatives, will be liable for damages arising out of or in connection with the use of this book.

You understand that this book is not intended as a substitute for consultation with a licensed healthcare practitioner. Before you begin any healthcare program, or change your lifestyle in any way, you should consult your physician or other licensed healthcare practitioner to ensure that you are in good health and that the examples contained in this book will not harm you.

Acknowledgement

I wish to acknowledge all of those men and women whom I have worked with over the years who helped me unravel the truth behind all of those wondrous and magical hormones that make us who we are. This book is dedicated to those of you who endured the suffering, who had the courage to seek out the truth, and who put their trust in my hands, including my daughter Amy, my wife Susan, and my sister Nancy. Without each of you, the rest of the world might have gone on to suffer needlessly. Thank you for daring to defy the status quo.

And a special note of gratitude to my wife Susan who unselfishly supported me and inspired me throughout the development of this book. Susan, you held me up when I faltered, you filled me with courage when I lost mine. Thank you, my earth angel.

Contents

Preface

When she walked into the office her eyelids were drooping. Her hair was thin and musty. Her skin color was that of plaster of Paris and carried a dull listless sheen. She sat down in the chair next to me, her lips parched and rigid. She had difficulty speaking to me but I got the message loud and clear. She didn't have to say a word. One look and I knew this sensitive woman was in the midst of a serious and disabling hormone crisis.

As a medical intuitive, I often sense or "know" what's going on before even one word is exchanged. Today was no exception. This forty-something peri-menopausal woman was literally lifeless, void of passion, inspiration, and of life force. I already knew that her libido was all but spent. I could sense that she had suffered from fibrocystic breasts and ovaries for many years. It was clear to me that she could barely summon up enough life energy to muster basic digestive and metabolic functions. She was alive, but that's as far as it went.

Sadly, this lovely woman had been in this dreadful state of basal existence for several years. Oh, yes, she had been compliant with her allopathic treatment regimen. She was taking estradiol for her hot flashes, yet the flashes still plagued her. She was faithfully indulging in levothyroxine for low thyroid function, and had been doing so for over ten years, yet her metabolic energy was mostly absent. She even dutifully followed the guidance of her primary care doctor when she instructed her to begin taking alendronate, a prescription medicine used to bolster low bone density, bone density that ironically eroded away through years of levothyroxine use.

Yes, this woman was the poster child of hormonally imbalanced women everywhere. The course of treatment she had been prescribed by her traditionally-trained gynecologist was convoluted and backwards and failed to address any of the underlying causes of these imbalances. As is all too common, the primary cause of hormone dysfunction had been overlooked and/or ignored by her mainstream gynecologist, endocrinologist, and primary care doctor. In fact, this "standard" traditional course of treatment used by tens of millions of hormonally imbalanced women around the globe often lead to the development of new health problems, not the least of which include chronic fatigue, loss of libido, mood swings, migraine headaches, high blood pressure, fibrocystic disease, and even hormonal cancers. It's almost as though every one of these women are being treated using the same cookbook; a cookbook filled with missing ingredients and misleading recipes.

Unfortunately, this wasn't the first time I'd seen this hormonal conundrum and it certainly wouldn't be the last. What I discovered over the years is that there was a crisis going on out there; a hormonal crisis that was seemingly ignored and misunderstood by the bulk of those operating under traditional medicine protocols. Hormonal complaints quickly became the number one issue among most every one of my clients, regardless of what these individuals believed they were coming to see me for originally, and despite having been under the care of hormonal specialists; their gynecologists and endocrinologists. Despite all these well-meaning practitioners and their cookbook treatment plans, things were not right.

Through my holistic methods, I would check the hormone levels of these individuals, and a trend quickly became apparent. Their hormones were out of balance, in many cases *way* out of balance, and these imbalances left 100% of these individuals with health repercussions that were not being attended to; health challenges so severe that many of these individuals were on the verge of suicide or developing cancer, or were just plain miserable. Yes, it became clear to me that traditional methods for managing the normal rhythm of hormonal shifts in men and women often left these individuals hormonally convoluted; literally left for dead.

It seems I had uncovered a hormonal pandemic, a bee's nest of hormonal horrors that over time brought many women to the brink of life system failure. Had I uncovered something no one else had seen? Was I examining aspects of the human make-up that others were not? Were traditional doctors simply not testing these individuals properly or were they failing to test the right things? Or was I just the last stop for the hormonally impaired train wrecks that no one else could balance? All of the above turned out to be true. I had uncovered an estrogen crisis.

I wrestled with all that I had learned and uncovered over those many years. I didn't know exactly what to make of it all, and I wasn't sure about how I wanted to handle the dissemination of these unique observations and findings, or if I even wanted to tackle the issue at all. After all, much of what I learned about hormone imbalances fully contradicted current practice guidelines, and would likely be considered unorthodox, unscientific, and even absurd by mainstream medicine practitioners who all learned something quite different from their medical school textbooks. My notions of hormonal management would fly in the face of everything traditional medical practitioners were told to believe. Was I ready or willing to be ridiculed, scoffed at, or simply ignored and viewed as some granola pharmacist quack?

Then one day out of the blue during the winter of 2010 the answer came in loud and clear. Yes. I *was* willing to risk it all; my reputation as a seasoned holistic healer and medical intuitive, my private practice in natural medicine. What good was any of it if I couldn't affect changes to improve the health and wellbeing of my fellow life journey partners? Somebody had to jar loose the massive cogwheels of what seemed to be a stagnant, narrow-focused healthcare system. And I got the assignment.

What follows is a fresh and unique perspective on the global hormonal crisis; a perspective beyond the science and beyond the pill protocols. It's a look through the eyes of a medical intuitive who is hell bent on getting to the true source of these hormonal miscues, taking you beyond the physical and the obvious, to a place that I sense is well beyond where healthcare has "advanced" thus far.

So prepare yourself for the journey. It may seem a little rocky at times as we navigate past the narrow and entrenched thinking of textbook modern medicine, as we challenge many of today's most staunch and time-honored notions about healthcare. But it's definitely worth the ride. It's a journey that will challenge you to look out of the box and help you realize there really is no box. *We* created the box. *We* created the limitations. And in this process we seem to have created false and dangerous misunderstandings, misguidance, and untruths about how best to manage our health. Now it's time to erase them all. Your health and survival may depend on it.

Emil Faithe
Albuquerque, NM
February 2013

Introduction

We are hormonal beings. Everything about us is controlled by our hormones. Our hormones control our mood, our sex drive, our energy levels, our level of excitement and alertness, the functionality of all of our organs, just about everything that makes us who we are. Even minute variations in our hormone levels can have a profound effect on how we feel physically, emotionally, spiritually, and mentally.

Each of us is born with a unique blend of hormones. It is this blend of hormones that dictates the type of person and personality we will express, and even the quality of living we will have in this lifetime. To be sure, our unique mix of each of the many hormones within us, defines us. This secret recipe of hormones that is unique to each of us is what makes us an individual and one-of-a-kind. Yes. *You* are one-of-a-kind.

We are comprised of many different kinds of hormones. These include hormones that control our kidney function and water balance, hormones like melatonin that controls our sleep state, or insulin that controls our blood sugar, and so many others. In this book we will be focusing our attention on the three key reproductive hormones, **progesterone, estrogen,** and **testosterone**. Why focus on the reproductive hormones? Because these three hormones control so many different physical and emotional aspects of ourselves, and because when out of balance, can have long reaching effects on nearly every other organ system in our body. In short, we will focus on progesterone, estrogen, and testosterone because from a health perspective they can either make you or break you. That is, day in and day out these three hormones can create more physical and emotional havoc and discomfort than any other, and almost always without our realizing it.

THE ATTENTION GRABBERS

These are also the same hormones that grab the most attention in the mass media. How many times have we endured the innuendos around women and their low estrogen levels, or painted a visual with a woman in PMS, premenstrual syndrome, holding a gun and demanding chocolate? These stereotypical behaviors are classical symptoms from the imbalance of these three notorious reproductive hormones.

And what would a women's life be like without the "curse" of menopause, that magical, mystical hormonal phase where a woman's entire being is turned upside down for all to see, again due to the carefully orchestrated re-alignment of progesterone, estrogen, and testosterone. Accompanied by the infamous hot flashes, this unique hormonal shift has certainly grabbed the attention of the beholder and hence the attention of health practitioners everywhere.

And as you'll learn, the male gender doesn't get a free pass either. Although garnering far less public attention, men most certainly do not escape the hormonal polar shifts unscathed either. We have our own "pause", one that I will refer to as andropause, or male menopause. Men experience their own unique set of concerns when it comes to reproductive hormone shifts, a shift that often leaves even the most macho man with fading libido, undiagnosed mood disorders, prostate dysfunction, and more.

Why progesterone, estrogen, and testosterone? Left unchecked, misalignment of these hormones both in men and women, can lead to serious health challenges including breast, uterine, and ovarian cancer in women, and prostate cancer in men, and leave both genders wondering what in the world hit them. And when all the current mainstream therapies fail to provide answers and relief, many will feel as though they've reached the end of their rope. Many will wonder if life is even worth living at all. Perhaps you are one of these individuals, or perhaps you know someone whose life has decayed into this hormonal rubble. If so, please do read on.

Is it any wonder then that these three powerful and misunderstood hormones, **progesterone, estrogen, and testosterone**, need such careful attention and nurturing? Is it any wonder why the time is *now* to uncover these hormone lies?

So where do we start? How do we go about uncovering the truth about these hormone misunderstandings? How do we get the attention of a world full of healthcare practitioners who have been programmed to view the hormones constellation one way, to begin looking at things in a whole *new* way? It starts by examining how hormone miscues have been managed in the past.

A BRAND NEW LOOK

There have been countless studies performed over the decades that discuss the minutia of hormone synthesis, degradation, the various pathways hormones are utilized, and modified, down-regulated and up-regulated, and all the rest of that scientific babble. But in my world there's more to healing an individual than all those equations, theorems, algorithms, and bar graphs on a sheet of paper. There's more to healing than the results of a blood test or a Pap smear. In this material we will voraciously avoid discussions that relate to specific blood levels, biological and chemical pathways, and all that other techno-science.

In fact, in this text we will steer clear of the mountains of scientific jargon and medical books and studies whose sole purpose is to provide scientific "proof" or "disproof" about all there is to know about hormones. We will stay clear of it simply because in truth, there really *is* nothing to prove. Some things just *are*, and can not be proven and need not be proven. Hormones and their actions are one of those things.

We're going to skip all that simply because as a medical intuitive I see the science as merely a morsel of the true health picture. There's more to see than meets the eye, and as a medical intuitive those unseen factors are what really matters. I'm interested in the energy fields of the organs, the emotional blocks that are disrupting physical and emotional harmony, the environmental exposures and genetics that are impacting your wellbeing, and more. Oh sure, we can not and should not forsake or discard science as a player in the healing process. Science has its place. But it also has its limitations. This material will help you decide when you've reached either.

In this book we're going to leave all that "proof" behind, simply because in this healer's opinion all that proof hasn't solved the problem. Too many individuals are still suffering despite all the science and technology, and *proof.* As the old and worn cliché goes, the proof is in the pudding, and I believe it's high time we all enjoy some pudding.

WHO MOVED THE PUDDING?

Why are we taking a fresh new look at the subject of hormone balance? Because the old look hasn't worked; because millions of women and men everywhere are still experiencing "unexplainable" and life-draining symptoms that are directly related to hormones that are not balanced. Hot flashes and the ravages of menopause and PMS still seem to confound mainstream health practitioners. The newly acknowledged hormonal chaos known as PCOS or Polycystic Ovary Syndrome, has literally gone viral among young females across the globe. Breast cancer, uterine, and ovarian cancer rates are climbing steadily despite all the research and world-wide fundraising in the name of curing it. Prostate cancer is now a new dreadful buzzword among men, young and old. To make matters even more intolerable, current treatment options offer little more than brutal, toxic, and costly sessions of chemotherapy, radiation, and surgery. You pick. Or rather, *they* pick.

Hormonally-induced mood swings, insomnia, anxiety, fatigue, and bone loss is at an all time high despite the use of expensive and toxic prescription medicines employed to treat them. Even more frightening, potent prescription estrogen replacement products are still being prescribed in the name of treating hormone imbalances, when in fact they are the root *cause* of many of the problems they are being used to treat, including endometriosis, fibrocystic breasts and ovaries, and hormonal cancers. And that's just for starters. When's it all going to stop? Something is amiss in the hormonal healing arena. In this book, we're going to uncover it.

Not only will we be taking a hard look at the way hormones affect literally every aspect of our life, you will be prompted to ask hard questions about any hormone intervention treatments before they begin, and you'll learn to understand why those questions need to be asked. You will discover new ways to balance your delicate hormones and the life issues they affect, without the need for potent prescription medicines. In essence, this material will help you simplify, demystify, and decode the hormone puzzle; the intrigue, all the cloak and dagger, so that you can separate the science from the fiction.

We will explore areas of hormone balancing that are almost never discussed with mainstream practitioners, and which lie at the heart of the silent global hormone crisis, including diet, nutrition, energy, emotions and more. We will pull open the curtain so you can see what's behind the hormone lies and thyroid misunderstandings. No, it's not Oz. It's the rainbow of help you've been searching for.

1.

Hormones: The Magical Messengers

We all have hormones. Hormones control our very existence. They play a crucial role in how we feel, how we behave, how we love, how we sleep, how we think… you name it. If we feel it, taste it, or sense it, there's a hormone behind it. But what are these unique chemical messengers that seem to affect so many aspects of us in such a profound way, each and every minute of every day? Are hormones these complex, mysterious, carbon-based materials with long, unpronounceable names, or are they something magical and indefinable?

Perhaps they are all of that. But rather than over-think the concept of hormones, maybe we should just accept the fact that hormones just *are*, accept them as a gift from Mother Nature; a gift of chemical messengers that defines us in every way. In this book, we're going to keep the concept of hormones wonderfully simple. Simple, so that we finally understand them; understand how they work, how they affect us, and how we can keep them in balance simply and easily. God knows, we don't need complicated. We already have enough of that in our lives.

HORMONES MADE SIMPLE

Let's do keep it simple. Let's imagine your hormones, any one of them, as powerful chemical messengers carrying very unique messages about yourself to all parts of your physical being. Think of them as text messages being sent from various organs and glands to literally any other organ and gland in the body. Hormones can send messages to the nervous system and affect our level of anxiousness, to the brain to make more of the hormone serotonin, the happy chemical, to the ovaries in women or the prostate in men to affect cell function there, or to the blood vessels that control our blood pressure. These chemical messengers literally criss-cross our entire physical makeup, affecting just about every bodily function, every emotion, every sensation we experience as beings.

Once the messages are received by the recipient organ, gland, or tissue, the recipient knows exactly what action to take to keep the physical body in proper balance. Now let's say these messages are sent incorrectly, maybe to the wrong recipient, or maybe there's too much information or not enough information in the chemical message, or the information or message is incomplete. It's these kinds of chemical message errors that can cause the recipient gland or organ to function incorrectly, creating undesirable actions, or what we know as "symptoms".

SIGNS AND SYMPTOMS OF PROGESTERONE, ESTROGEN, AND TESTOSTERONE IMBALANCES

- Weight disturbances
- Thyroid imbalances: hyper or hypo
- Depression
- Anxiety
- ADHD, Attention Deficit Hyperactivity Disorder
- Immune suppression
- Insomnia
- Headaches
- Candidiasis, Candida yeast infections
- Fatigue
- Increased pain perception
- Low libido or loss of "mojo"
- Hair growth
- Hair loss
- Difficult, painful, irregular periods
- Blood clots
- Pelvic pain
- Abnormal Pap smears or other negative cellular changes
- Skin changes, including acne
- Heart palpitations
- Endometriosis
- Tender breasts

- Low self-esteem
- Breakthrough bleeding
- Aggressiveness or edginess
- Fibrocystic breasts
- BPH, Benign Prostate Hypertrophy
- Ovarian cysts
- PCOS, Polycystic Ovary Syndrome
- Prostate cancer
- Ovarian cancer
- Breast cancer
- Uterine cancer
- Cholesterol imbalances
- Vocal range changes

This list of symptoms is not a comprehensive list by any means. Progesterone, estrogen, and testosterone imbalances can have a subtle or a profound impact on nearly every aspect of our physical, emotional and energetic wellness.

It's also important to note that many of the symptoms of progesterone, estrogen, testosterone imbalances listed above may be intensified and magnified in certain ultra-sensitive individuals. The opposite is also true; those with a stronger constitution may experience fewer symptoms or symptoms that are less intense. At the end of the day, the severity, intensity and duration of symptoms are ultimately determined by the genetic makeup, or the "inherent wiring" one was born with, and is also very much influenced by your nutritional and metabolic state at that particular moment in time.

No matter which angle you're looking from, hormone balance plays a vital role in our overall health and wellbeing. That is why it is so crucial to defend these hormones from anything that could disrupt their sensitive balance.

STAY CLEAR OF THE HORMONE MINE FIELDS

We live in a very challenging and energetically volatile world. So many powerful events are occurring all around us every minute of our day and across the globe. And each and every one of these events has the potential of having a negative impact on our delicate hormone profile; from the negativity of a television newscast, to the electronics we use day in and day out, to the energies of negative people we interact with. But that's just the beginning. Many other environmental elements can drag the sensitive individual through hormone hell.

It's become a well known fact that many of the pesticides sprayed onto the fruits and vegetables we consume each day are chemically similar to estrogen, hence mimic estrogen activity, and this estrogenic mimicking has led to a very real increase in the estrogen load in our environment and in our bodies. There are additional well-founded concerns with the plastic chemical byproduct BPA, bisphenol A, found in the plastic water bottles that millions of us drink from each day. Like estrogenic pesticides, this widely consumed chemical plasticizer can increase our estrogen load and under the right conditions lead to hormonal cancers. Just ask pop singer Sheryl Crowe. Drinking from hot bottled water containers for years was probably *not* one of her favorite mistakes. And the lists of chemicals that can disrupt estrogen go on and on. Clearly, these disruptors can be found anywhere in our environment and often in places we would never dream of. It's no wonder then that we are seeing alarming increases in breast cancer and other hormonal cancers, especially in women.

Hormone disruptors have a direct and profound effect on your hormone balance 24/7, even while you sleep and most often without your knowledge or permission. Yet, simply recognizing that these hormone minefields exist in your environment can provide you with the opportunity to step away from them, and help you protect your invisible magical messengers.

POTENTIAL HORMONE DISRUPTORS

- Past life trauma
- Post-traumatic stress disorder (PTSD) from rape, war, violence, accidents
- Over-nurturing others/under-nurturing self
- Any organ imbalance
- Menopause
- Andropause
- Illness of any kind
- Vaccinations of any kind

- Infections of any kind, including and especially Candidiasis
- Chemical exposures
- Surgery of any kind
- Stressful lifestyle
- Hysterectomy
- Birth control pills or devices
- Energy or entity attachments (a.k.a. ghosts)
- Prescription medicines
- Electromagnetic Field (EMF) emitters
  - cell phones/smart phones
  - computers
  - high voltage power lines
  - electric cars
  - x-rays
  - microwaves
  - televisions, especially digital devices
- Food ingredients and food allergies
- Harsh words
- Ley lines and energy vortexes of the planet
- Negative thinking
- Unhealthy relationships
- Lack of sexual expression
- Genetics
- Anger, resentment, guilt, shame, or any negative emotion

This list is far from comprehensive, since new disruptors are being discovered every day, many of them in the form of persons, places, and things you come into contact with every day. And no one is immune. Even individuals with the most stout of constitutions can be brought to their knees when enough hormone disruptors hit you at once. And they can.

KAREN is a 46-year old well-adjusted female with a relatively unremarkable upbringing. Oh sure, like all of us she had endured a few rough spots in her life journey, but nothing that shook her to her core—until the financial meltdown of 2008. A strong, confident woman, she had worked in corporate America for years and knew how to handle herself in most any situation. This was a woman in charge, yet a woman who balanced her life with calm, clear-headed thinking, and filled her spirit with inspiration and determination.

When she left the corporate world, she and her husband settled down and started a successful welding business and the money was flowing in. They shared a wonderful lifestyle together. They enjoyed plenty of vacations, built the home of their dreams, and enjoyed an active and rewarding sex life. All was well. Very well.

When Karen hit her early 40's she began to experience a few minor hormonal changes from the natural progression of menopause. An occasional hot flash would rear up and she seemed to lose some energy and stamina near the end of the day. But she experienced no severe or debilitating symptoms, until just weeks before we visited in my office in early 2011.

The real estate crash of 2008 created insidious and unforeseen stressors in Karen's life, which in turn caused her marriage of 18 years to hit some nasty snags. Her husband had become angry and distraught that their welding business was taking a dive, with business off by over 50 percent. The money wasn't flowing in any longer. In fact they where having a tough time managing the debt they took on during the more prosperous years.

Her husband became inconsolable and the typically strong and stout Karen was taking in all that negativity. Anger and resentment set in as each of them dealt the other a number of serious emotional blows. Not only that, the brand new home they recently downsized into was suddenly falling apart, and the builder was nowhere to be found. Their dream lifestyle was collapsing right in front of their eyes. Her relationship with her husband was also collapsing, with no end to the constant bickering in sight. Karen found herself in the middle of a financial and emotional collapse. The result: hormone hell.

Karen began to experience severe bouts of hot flashes, drenching her day and night. Her periods had suddenly become irregular and heavy, and what was once simply a small annoying breast cyst blossomed into full blown fibrocystic breast disease, with new and larger cysts appearing seemingly out of nowhere. Hair began falling out of her scalp in large clumps, creating serious self-esteem issues, and new hair growth was cropping above her lip and all over her face and other unwanted areas. When the panic attacks and insomnia set in, Karen knew something was seriously amiss. A friend referred her to my office.

I checked her hormones using applied kinesiology. Karen's emotional traumas had produced severely low progesterone levels and very high estrogen and testosterone levels, and this imbalance was directly responsible for her current physical and emotional state. The emotional stress had certainly taken a toll.

Karen started on a natural hormone balancing regimen I designed for her, that included topical progesterone cream, several natural estrogen modulators, and inositol to calm her mind and to balance her high testosterone levels. It took several months to get her hormones fully back to balance, but within three weeks many of her initial symptoms had begun to clear. Yet despite her visible progress it was obvious that Karen was still angry and resentful, and these negative emotions needed to be cleared in order to avert further hormonal disruptions.

After a series of emotional clearing sessions in my office, Karen seemed to become more comfortable within her own skin. Her facial expressions became more lax and natural. You could literally feel the blanket of calm and content exude itself. The anger and resentment she once harbored against her husband and the financial and legal system seemed to have completely disappeared. Oh sure, she had reason to be upset, but with her hormones now balanced she was able to handle these life stresses with nary a hitch. Yes, her marriage had ended, but amicably, and she soon began to take better care of herself, physically and emotionally. She began to eat healthy balanced meals, took up an exercising program and participated in a yoga class to help relieve the residual pent-up negativity. It worked.

Despite Karen's strong physical and emotional constitution, the great financial crash of 2008 had taken a toll, not just on Karen's bank account, but also on her hormonal balance. The hormone disruptors in her world took her by surprise, as they often do. But with a little help from a natural hormone replacement regimen and a sensible dose of energy and emotional clearing, Karen's life was back on track.

What Karen learned and what you can take from this case study is simply this: hormonal symptoms can be a powerful signal that something within us is not right. When interpreted as such, these discomforting symptoms can offer you a unique opportunity to make the necessary adjustments. This opportunity is nature's gift to you, and one that's best not ignored.

HORMONES: THEY DO A BODY GOOD

Hormones were part of the original design in the development of our species. They were designed to do the body good, and to do good things for the body, pleasurable things, to create harmony and balance in our lives, to give us the inspiration and desire to create and evolve, to supply the passion to procreate responsibly, and so much more. Yes, we are indeed hormonal beings.

Our hormones define us; they give us our identity. Without them we would be nothing more than a blank canvas in a meat suit. Hormones are nothing short of amazing messengers from our inner self, most literally from our genetic coding. When hormones are in balance they can provide us with feelings of bliss and euphoria, with pleasure and satisfaction, with drive and inspiration. But when out of balance they can send the human spirit, and the physical body within which it's housed, into a downward spiral of apathy, despair, and hopelessness.

Yes, our hormones can betray us if we let them. It makes sense then that we should evaluate the state of our hormone balance on a regular basis. Knowing where you stand hormonally not only gives you the tools to make any necessary changes, it also gives you an opportunity to take inventory of what's really taking place inside you, and not just at the physical level, but also at the emotional and energetic level. This knowledge won't be found in a blood test, x-ray, CAT scan, or in any medical book, yet it could be the most important thing you learn about yourself in this lifetime.

So spend a few moments and take your own hormone inventory. Once you do, you will have a much clearer sense as to why you may be experiencing some of the physical and emotional symptoms in your life. More importantly, you will have a better insight as to how to best apply the material presented in this book; information that can help you restore your natural balance, and propel you to your highest and best path for this lifetime.

TAKE THE HORMONE INVENTORY TEST

Circle ALL that apply:

1. Do you have resistant weight gain that won't budge no matter how much you exercise or how little you eat; especially around the waist, hips, or thighs? **PV = 4**
2. Do you suffer from frequent mood swings? **PV = 3**
3. Do you experience unexplainable hair loss or hair thinning? **PV = 2**
4. Is hair growing above your lip, on your face, your chest or back, or on any unwanted areas of your body? **PV = 3**
5. Have you always had or do you currently suffer from painful, unpredictable periods, with symptoms of bloating, edginess, and moodiness around your cycle dates? **PV = 4**
6. Do you always seem to get sick when others don't, or often have a "bug" of some sort? **PV = 1**
7. Have you been diagnosed with Polycystic Ovary Syndrome, or PCOS? **PV = 5**
8. Do you often feel fatigued, drained, listless, or even unproductive? **PV = 3**
9. Has your libido set sail for the Bahamas and left you with the bill? **PV = 4**
10. Do you find yourself snapping at others for no good reason? **PV = 3**
11. Are you experiencing difficulty falling asleep, staying asleep, or both, on a regular basis? **PV = 2**
12. Do you experience frequent headaches with no determinable cause? **PV = 3**
13. Have you been diagnosed with osteoporosis or osteopenia? **PV = 2**
14. Men, do you have difficulty urinating at any time of the day? **PV = 4**
15. Men, do you have difficulty achieving an erection? **PV = 4**
16. Has your vocal range recently dropped an octave or two? **PV = 3**
17. Are you experiencing bouts of rapid or skipped heart beats? **PV = 1**
18. Do you find yourself running out of steam early in the day? **PV = 2**
19. Do you suffer from regular bouts of apprehension, anxiety, or even panic attacks? **PV = 3**
20. Men, are your PSA (prostate-specific antigen) levels rising? **PV = 5**
21. Do you suffer from acne on your face, chest, or other areas of your body? **PV = 3**
22. Do you often feel weepy and melancholy? **PV = 3**

23. Do you feel as though you can't cope with the world, or that the world is overwhelming to you? **PV = 3**
24. Do you experience regular vaginal dryness or painful intercourse **PV = 2**
25. Do you have fibrocystic breasts, or experience regular breast tenderness or "lumpiness"? **PV = 4**
26. Have you had an abnormal Pap exam, or been diagnosed with pre-cancerous cellular changes in your reproductive organs? **PV = 5**
27. Do you often experience hot flashes or night sweats? **PV = 3**
28. Are you taking prescription estrogen or progesterone medicines, including birth control? **PV = 4**
29. Are you experiencing memory loss, mental confusion, or difficulty concentrating?
PV = 2
30. Do you have frequent bouts of vaginal yeast infections? **PV = 1**
31. Have you been diagnosed with endometriosis? **PV = 4**
32. Do you experience sharp pain or any pain in your pelvic area during or around your period, whether you still have one or not? **PV = 5**

PV stands for point value. Total the point value of each of the phrases that best describes your situation. If your total point value is between:

WOMEN

0 to 10 points - No clinically significant hormone disruptions have yet occurred, but they could start at any time. Pay close attention to any further symptoms that may arise.

10 to 20 points - Your hormones are in the process of shifting and the progress of the shift may not have reached its peak. This hormone shift may be due to the natural life cycle we call menopause, and this is more likely the case if you are between the ages of 35 and 60. If under age 35, look for possible hormonal disruptors that may be in play in your life and get your hormones and your lifestyle evaluated by a qualified holistic practitioner.

20 to 40 points - A potent and disruptive hormone shift is definitely in progress and needs to be closely monitored to prevent unwanted physical and emotional symptoms from accelerating. At this stage your body is giving you very definite signs and signals that something is amiss and needs your prompt attention. It's time to take a much closer and harder look at all the hormone disruptors in your life, including unhealthy relationships, hormonal prescriptions (including birth control), and hysterectomies that are not accompanied by progesterone supplementation. Get your hormone profile evaluated with your chosen practitioner promptly to avoid organ damage and any further disruption of the joy in your life.

40 points or more - Your estrogen to progesterone ratio and your overall hormone balance is dangerously out of balance. Cell and organ damage has likely begun and will likely progress unless and until an intervention occurs. At this stage, life is generally unpleasant, and you may be experiencing significant deterioration of energy levels, loss of libido, insomnia, and a general malaise; in a nutshell, your life may be quite miserable. If this hormone imbalance is not attended to promptly, you are at risk of developing negative cellular changes including hormonal cancers, especially if there is any family history of the same. A visit with a qualified holistic practitioner is most definitely warranted as soon as possible. Do not delay.

MEN

0 to 10 points - No clinically significant hormone disruptions have yet occurred, but they could start at any time. Pay close attention to any further symptoms that may arise.

10 to 20 points - your hormone balance is in the midst of a shift I call andropause, or male menopause, and this occurs quite commonly between the ages of 40 and 60. Although the symptoms of andropause often go unrecognized, and are certainly less talked about, it is a male life event that is quite real. At this stage it would not be uncommon to experience lower moods, lower energy and stamina, and a fading libido. Consult with a practitioner if these symptoms do not improve with proper dietary changes, namely increasing protein consumption, and lifestyle changes which should include reducing stress levels and rethinking work and life productivity expectations.

20 points or more - Significant hormonal disruption has likely peaked or is about to peak and these changes may be wreaking havoc on your heart health, stamina, and overall life experience. You may also be experiencing conflicts in many if not all of your relationships. As well, negative cellular changes may be in progress, to the point of causing BPH, benign prostate hypertrophy, or an enlargement of the prostate, even prostate cancer. These symptoms tend to be more prominent in sensitive men, and there are plenty of you out there, despite your size and your station in life. Schedule a visit with your qualified holistic practitioner to evaluate your hormone profile. Don't be ashamed or embarrassed to express your feelings and emotions, and do discuss all of your issues candidly, both with your partner and your practitioner.

NO NEED TO PANIC

If you didn't score well in the Hormone Inventory Test, don't fret. You are not alone. Tens of millions of women and men across the globe are living with important hormonal imbalances and in many cases have been doing so for years, even decades. What's worse, most of these individuals have no idea that their hormone imbalance may be causing the symptoms they have been living with. But now *you* do. You're eons ahead of most everybody out there. That's what this book is all about. Uncovering the truth about progesterone, estrogen, and testosterone imbalances and teaching you how to piece together your own hormone puzzle and in the process; solving your personal health puzzle. It's about uncovering the hormone lies and thyroid misunderstandings.

IS IT TOO LATE FOR ME?

It's never too late to correct hormone imbalances. When recognized early, these hormone miscues and the negative effects they have caused can often be fully corrected using sensible holistic and natural means. It may take several months or longer to accomplish this task, but that time frame is negligible when you consider the fact that these imbalances have developed slowly and insidiously over decades, often over your entire lifetime.

For this reason, I encourage you to continue reading through the material in this book so that you can find solutions to the hormone conundrums you are experiencing right now. Once you're done, you will have much of the information you need to take positive action. So please do give those magical chemical messengers we call "hormones" the care and attention they deserve. Why? Because they are an intrinsic part of *you*; they define you. And you and your hormones deserve nothing short of balance, bliss, and wellbeing.

2.

Classic Hormonal Miscues Decoded

Depression
Anxiety
Insomnia
Fibrocystic Breasts and Ovaries
Weight Gain
Low Libido
Hot Flashes

Hormones control everything we're about. When they're in balance they can make us feel good; elated, amorous, tranquil, energetic, inspired, content, and balanced in every way. When they're out of balance those same hormones can make us feel simply miserable, depressed, anxious, hopeless, exhausted and listless, and can send our health into a dismal downward spiral. Which set of descriptors would you rather experience in *your* lifetime? – I thought so.

But as we have seen, many factors in our daily lives can alter our delicate and unique hormone balance of progesterone, estrogen, and testosterone, and when they do, some of the most prevalent, uncomfortable, dreaded health challenges can rear their ugly heads. But we can prevent all that by simply looking at the hormone platform in a whole new way. In doing so, you have the opportunity to learn the truth about what makes your hormones tick, and about the kind of care and feeding they've been longing for.

HORMONE LIES

No more pharmaceutical agendas. No more knee-jerk, blinders-on treatment of hormone challenges. No more text-book, science-is-king thinking. We're taking a hard new look at the common progesterone, estrogen, and testosterone-induced health maladies, those health challenges you or your loved ones are likely still dealing with on a daily basis. Endometriosis, fibrocystic breast disease, PCOS, loss of libido, and fatigue, and that's just before you get up in the morning. It's time for a change and some real results, not just a cover-up, spearheaded by a pill or a patch.

Am I out to start a hormone revolution? Maybe. Am I writing this material in an attempt to aggravate those who see things differently than I, or to bash those who embrace the status quo in hormone treatment? That's certainly not my intention. Regardless, a great many practitioners trained by the traditional medical system will likely balk at my findings, notions, and concepts. They will vehemently declare them unorthodox, too simplified and lacking in scientific studies, "Where is the proof?" they will cry. I have no proof, I only have results, results in thousands of women and men who have been down the path of traditional hormone balancing regimens only to find themselves at their wits end, still suffering and using countless pills and patches in an attempt to improve their lives. Yet in too many cases they were no better off than they were before they started these various treatment regimens and in many cases they were worse, much worse.

I have been successful in helping these individuals because I took my blinders off, and I listened carefully, observed even more carefully, and I checked and determined through my holistic means the true causes of the symptoms that were presented before me. And after 30 years of careful listening, observation, and holistic treatment with methods that might be considered unconventional by some, these individuals finally got better. That's *my* proof. And that's what's in this book.

So for those who need other types of proof, please seek out the medical libraries online where you may find the studies you so crave. As for me, I'm simply a medical intuitive, venturing out of the bounds and out of the shackles of science in an attempt to bring relief to the millions who suffer despite the best efforts of modern medicine.

If you are reading this book, you or someone you love is likely one of those still suffering from hormonal chaos I am about to unveil, or at the very least one of those who is ready for a real change. So let's start by examining the current state of the hormone treatment dilemma.

HORMONE TRUTH #1

Not enough practitioners are paying attention to the key signs and signals of hormone imbalances. Many obvious clues are being overlooked or ignored.

HORMONE TRUTH #2

The testing methods used to check for hormone imbalances are not always accurate or representative of the whole hormone picture.

HORMONE TRUTH #3

The results of these tests are not correctly interpreted within context of the overall clinical picture. Treatment plans based on these results do not address the underlying causes of the symptoms presented.

HORMONE TRUTH #4

Current treatment methods focus only on a limited and antiquated arsenal of toxic and obtrusive prescription pills or patches, which often bring on new symptoms and aggravate the underlying cause.

IT'S GOOD TO KNOW

Now that we've identified the dilemma, let's begin to explore the solutions.

The material that follows has been assembled in a simple, matter-of-fact style, designed to hit you "right between the eyes". That's because I have found that understanding and managing hormone imbalances does not have to be complicated. Decoding and balancing hormones doesn't have to be shrouded in mystery as many might like you to believe. At the end of the day what really matters is that what you learn from this book helps bring you a higher quality of living, that it makes you feel better than you did before you set out reading this book. If that is what you take away from this, then I have done my job well.

With that in mind, let's take a closer look at the top hormonal maladies and their remedies as seen through the eyes of a medical intuitive, one at a time.

Depression

LOW PROGESTERONE CAN LEAD TO DEPRESSION

By my gauge, the health condition we know as depression has become today's modern plague. Accompanied by its all too familiar cohorts despair, sadness and apprehension, depression has decimated the joy in the lives of countless individuals across the globe. It is estimated that over 25 million Americans and over 120 million people worldwide suffer from the emotional/physical syndrome the medical community calls "depression". Based on my experience working with a cross section of the population, I would suggest those numbers are grossly under-reported. One way or another, depression seems to have taken a serious foothold among the fabric of our society.

And while many factors can lead to the onset of this disabling malady, including mercury and other heavy metal toxicities, Candidiasis, and poor nutrition, it is the imbalances in progesterone, estrogen, and testosterone that are almost always overlooked as a culprit. Yet ironically, hormone imbalances are often the underlying cause of depression, especially among the female gender. This is borne out by the fact that an astounding *70 percent* of all those afflicted by depression are female.

That statistic alone should be enough to raise a red flag in the minds of the traditional doctors who are faced with symptoms of depression in their female patients. But most often it does not. In most cases, traditional practitioners simply never put two and two together, and hormone rebalancing is never considered for the purpose of resolving depression. Instead, women become just another statistic, and the recipient of the latest and greatest antidepressant medication.

Sadly, today's modern medicine fails to ask the question "why is my patient depressed?" If they *had* asked, and followed through with a proper and thorough investigation they would likely discover that there are a number of factors that should be considered in solving the mood pandemic, many of them under our nose and in our everyday life. One of those factors is low progesterone.

COMMONLY OVERLOOKED CAUSES OF DEPRESSION

- Candidiasis, Candida yeast infections
- Energy or entity attachments (a.k.a. ghosts)
- Viral infections
- Hypoglycemia
- Malnutrition, especially protein deficiency
- Genetic ultra-sensitivity
- Toxic exposures
- Lack of sexual expression
- Hysterectomy
- Food ingredients and food allergies
- Relationship and social stress including unbalanced family dynamics
- Post-traumatic stress disorder (PTSD) from any life event, current or past life
- Prescription medicines including birth control
- **Low progesterone**

LOOKING IN ALL THE WRONG PLACES

As you can see there are a number of easily correctable factors in your life that may be responsible for your low mood. These commonly overlooked culprits are likely in your life right now, and most have likely never been addressed by anyone. Low progesterone levels are one of them.

Low progesterone levels over time will lead to low serotonin levels and low serotonin is the key brain chemical responsible for low mood, appetite changes, weight gain, sleep disturbances, and more. As such, when progesterone levels are supplemented through a topical application and brought back to balance, these symptoms will often resolve over a three to six month period, and without the need for prescription antidepressants. Sure, prescription antidepressants may improve some symptoms for some individuals, but ultimately these harsh medicines often cause new problems. One of those problems is sexual dysfunction, an unwanted side effect that is equally devastating to both men and women. Ironically, if progesterone levels had been corrected in the first place, libido and sexual function would be restored through gentle and natural means, the way nature intended. The progesterone/depression connection is a hormonal conundrum indeed.

17

The message is simple. If you are a woman between the ages of twelve and infinity and are suffering from the symptoms of depression, *any of them*, get your hormones checked and balanced through natural means without delay.

SOONER THAN LATER

Most individuals believe that significant hormonal shifts only occur during those hormonally-transitional years in a woman's life cycle called menopause, typically during their 40's or 50's. Nothing could be further from the truth. Hormone imbalances can begin at any age, often at puberty, and even from the womb, if genetics have their way. That's why it is important to consider low progesterone as the cause for any physical and emotional health challenges regardless of age, and this holds especially true for the constellation of symptoms we call depression. And because the new crop of young beings coming in now tend to be exceptionally sensitive, or what I call *ultra-sensitive*, hormone disruption, and any organ disruption for that matter, can occur much more readily and have more devastating physical and emotional consequences than ever before.

Unfortunately, the traditional medical community hasn't embraced that possibility when it comes to managing the health issues of young beings. As a result we are seeing young women and men, being subjected to toxic antidepressant medicines like fluoxetine, paroxetine, sertraline, buproprion — even medicines to treat attention deficit (an absurd term) with medicines like methylphenidate, amphetamine and dextroamphetamine salts, and atomoxetine — even in young people ages five and up! There's nothing more disturbing to an ultra-sensitive medical intuitive than to witness a six-year old taking fluoxetine for mood or anxiety issues. And I have indeed seen this on too many occasions.

RACHEL is a very gifted, very sensitive 14-year old who was referred to my office by her mother for her persistent mood swings. Her mother, a holistic healer in her own right, was concerned that her usual attempts to improve her daughter's mood had failed.

Just seconds into our visit, it became clear to me that we were dealing with a sensitive and an exceptionally gifted soul. This young being was definitely connected to other dimensions, and not always present in this one, which is quite often the case in ultra-sensitive individuals. Her affect was quite subdued, and she initially appeared very shy and reserved with me. After putting her at ease, I tuned-in and asked my usual set of probing questions.

As it turns out, Rachel's diet was actually quite appropriate, and her social and lifestyle factors all seemed to be quite reasonable and in order. Fortunately her holistic-minded mother had the foresight to avoid prescription medicines in this situation, since those would have likely made matters worse. Her mother did however start Rachel on several natural and gentle mood elevators, but in this case the B vitamins and fish oil had no effect on young Rachel's mood.

I took the opportunity to open the conversation up to more eclectic topics and that's when Rachel's eyes popped open with intrigue. This was not your average 14-year old. Rachel had a deep and mature understanding of herself and her place in this world. She expressed a keen interest and understanding of energy and metaphysics, which is quite typical for these special beings. Once her mother agreed to leave the room for a moment, Rachel also confided that she had a difficult time relating to those around her, including the kids in her school, and even her siblings and her parental unit. She also reported that her period had begun and that they had been painful and irregular.

That was enough proof for me. I immediately started Rachel on a hormone and mood balancing regimen that included low-dose progesterone cream and a whey protein shake to help build and strengthen her serotonin balance. A bit chagrined at first, her mother agreed to give it a try. Within three months Rachel's mood had become noticeably brighter, she had become less anxious and more inspired, and her periods had begun to normalize. Eight months later her mother reported that all was back to normal.

As for Rachel's profound sensitivity and knowing, well her mother asked that I work with Rachel to help cultivate and guide her gifted daughter's spiritual prowess. Few things please me more than to assist a young being on their path of ultra-sensitivity. It was certainly my pleasure to work with such a connected and gifted individual. It was even more rewarding to have been able to correct a simple hormonal imbalance in order to help bring flight to such a special soul.

MIXED SIGNALS

In most cases, the need for progesterone supplementation is quite obvious. Correct the low progesterone levels and off they go, happily ever after. However, now and again, it takes a bit more than simple progesterone supplementation to make things right; more often than not it requires keen observation and a king-size dose of intuition to solve the hormone puzzle. That means exploring the *less* obvious signs and signals that a hormone deficiency may be at play. That's why it's imperative to examine the whole clinical picture and all the issues at play in the life of an individual to solve what some traditional practitioners often refer to as "medical mysteries". For me, there are no such things. There's always a reason and always a cause. You just have to know how and where to look for it. After 30 years of finding the pieces of these puzzles, Julie's case was no exception.

JULIE is a delightful peri-menopausal woman who came to see me because of extreme mood swings she had been dealing with for the past year. She reported that her moods had always been quite stable and that she was generally a very happy person, hence these new feelings of sadness, hopelessness, and negativity came as quite an unpleasant surprise to her. Working hard to stay clear of the knee-jerk antidepressant prescription mill, Julie had tried several natural antidepressant formulas containing St. John's wort prior to seeing me, but those produced little results.

Our first few minutes together were a bit confounding. Julie had none of the usual hormonal suspects that one would expect to see during the menopausal shift. She was not overweight, her sleep was generally restful, and she complained of only rare and mild hot flashes. Even libido seemed quite balanced. But first glances are sometimes deceiving if you're not looking at the whole clinical picture, and if you haven't taken the opportunity to "pull back the curtain". I did. It turns out that Julie's siblings and most of her female relatives on both sides of her family suffered from fibrocystic breasts, breast cancer scares, and yes, mood issues. Nearly every one of her female relatives suffered from late-life mood disturbances, and Julie was following in the footsteps of her genetic lineage all too closely.

When I checked her hormones through kinesiology, I had expected to find substantially low progesterone levels and high estrogen levels. What I found instead was that her progesterone levels were only *slightly* low, in my experience not typically low enough to illicit mood issues. Yes, her estrogen levels were high as I sensed they would be, and estrogen dominance was the genesis behind the ancestral cystic and pre-cancerous cell changes in her genetic lineage. But I followed my hunch and we started topical progesterone cream anyway. My other sense about Julie is that she was harboring a raging Candida infection, a yeast infection, and that infection was most definitely contributing to her low mood as well. Systemic Candida infections, or Candidiasis, are notorious for causing depression in sensitive individuals. That was Julie.

Within eight weeks of topical progesterone treatment and a Candida-fighting regimen, Julie's depressive symptoms completely disappeared one day, almost as quickly as they appeared. I encouraged Julie to continue the progesterone regimen I had laid out, albeit at a lower dose, to maintain the progesterone balance we had achieved. And because Julie was an energy worker and an empath, one who easily feels the energies of everybody and everything, I cautioned her to protect herself more carefully when working with her clients, many of whom were dealing with their own mood and hormone imbalances. She got the message.

Last we connected Julie was still symptom-free and to boot, was not experiencing *any* of the typical menopausal symptoms. This was the blessing that she had hoped for, and I had wished for her, and wishes *do* come true.

In this case, the symptoms of estrogen imbalance were quite obvious, yet the symptoms of low *progesterone* were more elusive. In the end, all of the puzzle pieces fit neatly into place. And that's the way I like it.

MOOD MAGIC

Supplementing with topical progesterone cream isn't always the only fix for sagging mood issues, but it almost always plays some role in resolving mood issues, especially in females. For that reason, it's important to visit with a qualified holistic practitioner versed in natural hormone replacement to check your hormone level using applied kinesiology. When properly accomplished, your practitioner should be able to connect all the dots and develop a treatment protocol to balance your mood naturally.

HORMONE TRUTH:

If you suffer from the symptoms of depression, progesterone levels should be checked and balanced before any other interventions are begun.

HORMONE BALANCING REGIMEN FOR DEPRESSION

For women still cycling:

Topical progesterone cream ¼ to ½ teaspoonfuls rubbed into breast, stomach, thighs, or inner arm once daily at bedtime on your cycle days 12 through 26. The first day of your cycle is the first day of bleeding.

For women no longer cycling:

Topical progesterone cream ¼ to ½ teaspoonfuls rubbed into breast, stomach, thighs, or inner arm once daily at bedtime on calendar days 1 through 25 only.

- Rotate application site every two to three days
- It may take two to three months or longer to notice full improvement of symptoms, so be patient
- Hormone levels should be checked through applied kinesiology throughout the balancing period at approximately three to four week intervals

Anxiety

LOW PROGESTERONE AND HIGH ESTROGEN AND
TESTOSTERONE CAN LEAD TO ANXIETY

Anxiety. Just the word alone conjures up squirmy feelings in most individuals. Heart racing, profuse sweating, chest and throat tightening, knees knocking… anxiety in its various forms and various degrees plagues millions of individuals everywhere. It is said to be the most common "mental illness" in America, affecting upward of 50 million people, and climbing. Clearly those who experience anxiety at any level can attest to the fact that the symptoms of anxiety are uncomfortable at best and for many disabling, making for a very unpleasant life journey and sucking the joy out of all of life's pleasantries.

The sensations of anxiety can range from mild feelings of restlessness, to constant low-level apprehension, to full-blown panic attacks, and beyond. No matter how you slice it or dice it, anxiety is no one's friend. If you or someone you know suffers from the ravages of anxiety this is not news to you.

Most individuals will peg the blame of anxiety, fear, and apprehension we experience on all the stressors in our society, the more tangible aspects of our lives; stresses in our relationships, money challenges, the rigors of our careers or our jobs. Make no mistake, these life challenges can indeed have a negative impact on our balanced nature, yet I would suggest that there are a number of other factors that create anxiety in our lives that most never even consider.

Here is a list of those less-obvious culprits that may be behind your state of uneasiness; those hidden, less tangible disruptors of the calm that can shake even the most stout individuals in their tracks; anxiety inducers likely you and your health practitioner may have never considered, or just simply overlooked.

COMMONLY OVERLOOKED CAUSES OF ANXIETY

- Candidiasis, Candida yeast infection
- Hypoglycemia
- Malnutrition, especially protein deficiency
- Genetic ultra-sensitivity
- Food ingredients and food allergies
- Iodine deficiency
- Protein deficiency
- Relationship and social stress including unbalanced family dynamics
- Prescription medicines including birth control
- Electromagnetic Field (EMF) emitters
  - cell phones/smart phones
  - computers
  - high voltage power lines
  - electric cars
  - x-rays
  - microwaves
  - televisions, especially digital devices
- Energy or entity attachments (a.k.a. ghosts)
- Lack of sexual expression
- Hysterectomy
- Post-traumatic stress disorder (PTSD) from any life trauma, current or past life
- **Low progesterone**
- **High estrogen**
- **High testosterone**

IT'S OUT THERE

We live in a fast-paced world, a world where instant gratification - "what else you got?", "I need more input!" - *rules*. Everything you want to know, everything you want to hear, everything you want to see, literally everything you want to *have* is now available at the tips of your fingers with the ever-evolving "smart phones." We are constantly bombarded with things to do and things to think about. Today, the world is open 24/7. It's no wonder then that anxiety and its cousins, apprehension and fear, are on a meteoric rise on this planet. Maybe all that input isn't so smart after all.

And when it comes to hormone disruption, there are no maybes about it. This barrage of energetic and electronic input can quickly and easily disrupt any bodily function, and any hormone balance, and especially progesterone, estrogen, and testosterone levels. And when these three important hormones find an *un*happy balance, anxiety is sure to follow. And that unhappy balance looks like this:

LOW progesterone plus HIGH estrogen plus HIGH testosterone = ANXIETY

Does this theorem hold true? In my experience the answer is absolutely yes. When a natural regimen designed to raise progesterone and lower estrogen and testosterone is instituted, anxiety levels will subside in the majority of cases over a two to three month period, often sooner. And when it comes to managing anxiety and apprehension, it's always nice to get an extra boost from a welcome friend, protein.

PUNCH IT UP

Even though bringing progesterone, estrogen, and testosterone into balance is key to curbing anxiety, two important and seemingly overlooked nutritional deficiencies seem to stand out as accomplices in the anxiety conundrum, and should also be addressed at the same time progesterone cream is introduced.

Supplementing with amino acids in the form of dietary protein can be extremely helpful in clearing the uneasiness you may be feeling. Why protein? Protein is made up of the amino acids that are used to manufacture powerful anxiety-balancing neurochemicals; brain chemicals like serotonin, GABA or gamma amino butyric acid, a key calming neurotransmitter and other chemicals involved in maintaining the calm. And despite your dress or pant size and what most practitioners and others may believe, most everyone is protein deficient and usually without realizing they are.

Supplementing your diet with a whey protein shake daily is a great place to start. This should be accompanied by additional protein intake in the form of turkey, chicken, beef, eggs, fish, beans, nuts and seeds. Protein food stuffs should be a part of each of at least three properly-spaced meals, and up to six smaller meals throughout the day. In fact, protein "grazing" is actually quite a healthy practice and one that is not practiced enough. Why should you eat protein more frequently throughout the day? This frequent exposure to protein not only helps kick up the production of those key neurotransmitters responsible for keeping anxiety in check, it also helps reduce bouts of hypoglycemia, another powerful trigger of anxiety, apprehension, and low mood.

Iodine supplementation is another highly overlooked yet vital ally in the fight against anxiety and apprehension, yet traditional practitioners almost never consider low iodine levels as a cause of anxiety and almost never check iodine levels. Yet low levels of this key nutrient can quietly and insidiously wreak havoc not just in the female world, but is especially important in easing chronic anxiety in anxious males everywhere. A qualified holistic practitioner can remedy that situation by checking and balancing iodine using applied kinesiology techniques. Once iodine levels are corrected, long-standing feelings of apprehension, anxiety, and fear will often melt away over a short period of time. You can explore more about this phenomenon in the Iodine chapter.

The battle against anxiety is often one fought on several fronts, yet righting the balance between progesterone, estrogen, and testosterone is vital in solving the anxiety puzzle. And given the emotional and physical toll that anxiety and fear takes on the lives of countless millions, who suffer mostly in silence, it's a battle worth fighting.

TATIANA is a gentle and compassionate fifty-something woman who appeared in my office complaining of new-onset anxiety. It didn't take but a moment for me to realize the reason for her visit on this mild fall day; she was squirming in her chair, tapping her fingers and her toes as though listening to a concert in her head, and her speech had a discernable stutter. You could almost hear her teeth clattering as she wiped away a falling tear. Being an empath, I needed to shield myself from the powerful waves of anxiety I was feeling; as her feelings of squirminess and anxiousness quickly became my feelings of squirminess and anxiousness. Something had to be done quickly; otherwise both of us were at risk of going into a full blown panic attack.

I wasted no time. I asked Tatiana to take an inositol capsule I keep available for cases like this. A safe B vitamin, inositol would rapidly help lower what I sensed were Tatiana's high, very high testosterone levels. When I returned ten minutes later she had calmed noticeably and we were able to proceed with our investigation into her symptoms of extreme anxiety.

Tatiana's history was generally unremarkable. She was taking only a B vitamin complex, was taking no prescription medications, and reported no traumatic events in her life save for the usual childhood emotional bumps and bruises. She did however reveal that these waves of anxiety commenced immediately after a near-miss car accident three months earlier. This was an important fact, since physical and emotional trauma, or PTSD, is a potent anxiety trigger that can rear itself almost instantaneously.

Her hormone history was also unremarkable, except that unlike many women in her age group, Tatiana had not encountered any of the usual hormonal symptoms during her menopausal journey. Like her mother, she never had to deal with hot flashes, difficult periods, loss of libido, or weight issues. In fact, her weight was perfect for her five-foot three-inch frame. I had found over the years that this sort of genetic blessing occurs in a fortunate 10 to 15 percent of the female population, yet just because she did have the typical physical and emotional symptoms did not necessarily mean that all of Tatiana's hormones were in balance. For that reason I proceeded to conduct a complete hormone check in the usual fashion, using applied kinesiology.

What I found first surprised me, but then the puzzle pieces once again fell into place. Tatiana presented with just slightly low progesterone levels and *normal* estrogen levels, quite a rare occurrence in this age group, and that finding accounted for her lack of hot flashes. But the real culprit behind all her sudden angst also became clear. As I had sensed earlier, her testosterone levels were extremely high, so high in fact that her thyroid function kicked into high gear and was raging. Tatiana was in a temporary but very real *hyper*thyroid state, and she was most definitely feeling the rev.

The verdict: A combination of low progesterone from family genetics and high testosterone due to her post traumatic near-miss car crash were the triggers behind Tatiana's state of anxiety. This conclusion also triggered an "ah hah" moment for Tatiana. She confessed that her symptoms of anxiety always seemed worse after traveling in a car, either as the driver or the passenger. In fact, she admitted with some embarrassment that the drive over to my office triggered her initial jittery presentation. I worked to ease her feelings of embarrassment and went on to suggest that her anxiety symptoms could be controlled with a natural hormone balancing regimen. She insisted upon it immediately and I was happy to comply.

After only two days of taking inositol four times a day and applying a ¼ teaspoonful dose of topical progesterone cream daily per my instruction, Tatiana's anxiety symptoms began to subside dramatically, so much so, she made a point of driving herself over for the first time since her automobile incident, for our one-week follow-up to share the good news. Her car phobias had all but disappeared and her anxiety levels had dropped from a nine out of ten to a two out of ten, a huge improvement. And it showed. Tatiana looked and felt like a new woman; calm, controlled, this time smiling without any teeth clattering.

ABOLISH ANXIETY

Anxiety is without a doubt one of the most uncomfortable, joy-sucking events that can occur to a being on this planet. If you don't suffer from these nasty symptoms, count your blessings. If you are one of the tens of millions who do, or know someone who does, rest assured that a proper natural hormone balancing regimen instituted under the guidance of a qualified health practitioner can often be all that is needed to restore calm and contentment in your life. You too can abolish anxiety naturally.

HORMONE TRUTH:

If you suffer from the symptoms of anxiety, testosterone and progesterone levels must be carefully checked and balanced and should be augmented with adequate protein intake, and iodine when necessary.

HORMONE BALANCING REGIMEN FOR ANXIETY

1. Progesterone cream

For women still cycling:

Topical progesterone cream ¼ to ½ teaspoonfuls rubbed into breast, stomach, thighs, or inner arm once daily at bedtime on your cycle days 12 through 26. The first day of your cycle is the first day of bleeding.

<u>For women no longer cycling:</u>

Topical progesterone cream ¼ to ½ teaspoonfuls rubbed into breast, stomach, thighs, or inner arm once daily at bedtime on calendar days 1 through 25 only.

- Rotate application site every two to three days
- It may take two to three months or longer to notice full improvement of symptoms, so be patient
- Hormone levels should be checked through applied kinesiology throughout the balancing period at approximately three to four week intervals

2. Inositol 500 to 2000mg orally up to four times daily as needed for feelings of anxiety or apprehension.

- Do not exceed daily doses of 10,000mg daily without guidance
- May cause excess drowsiness in higher doses in sensitive individuals. Use the lowest effective dose
- Inositol is not addictive and may be used on a continuous basis indefinitely
- Inositol has no significant interactions with any prescription medicines

3. Iodine 150 to 300mcg once daily in the morning at least ½ hour before food.

- Higher doses may be required in some cases. Do not exceed the above doses without professional guidance
- Although true iodine allergies are quite rare, do not take supplemental iodine without guidance if you have a documented allergy to iodine
- Iodine levels should be checked through applied kinesiology throughout the balancing period at approximately three to four week intervals

4. Whey protein shake: one serving in almond milk or other non-dairy milk or water for breakfast in *addition* to breakfast food. May take an additional serving at about 2pm daily

- If you are a vegetarian, you may substitute a vegetarian protein shake in place of whey, and this practice is highly encouraged

Insomnia

LOW PROGESTERONE CAN LEAD TO INSOMNIA

Got sleep? For over 30 million Americans the answer is simply NO. Insomnia is one of the most under-rated and *under-treated* health problems in the world. Under-treated because the medical community's answer for sleeplessness is to force your organs to sleep with harsh, habit forming pills, rather than fixing the underlying problem. And if you're not sleeping, you're simply not living well. That's because sleep deprivation can lead to some serious and chronic health problems including weight gain, cancer, heart disease, immune issues, blood sugar problems, and that's just for starters.

If you're not getting seven to nine hours of quality REM, rapid eye movement sleep, you're setting yourself up for an unhappy and unproductive life experience.

COMMONLY OVERLOOKED CAUSES OF INSOMNIA

- Hypoglycemia
- Food ingredients and food allergies
- Genetic ultra-sensitivity to planetary energies
- Protein deficiency
- Hysterectomy
- Hot flashes
- Prescription medicines including birth control
- Post-traumatic stress disorder (PTSD) from any life trauma, current or past life
- Electromagnetic Field (EMF) emitters
  - cell phones/smart phones
  - computers
  - high voltage power lines
  - electric cars
  - x-rays
  - microwaves
  - televisions, especially digital devices

- Energy or entity attachments (a.k.a. ghosts)
- **Low progesterone levels**

TOO MUCH INPUT

Insomnia is a complex health challenge. It has many causes and truly many solutions, many of which are never recognized or addressed. First and foremost it is important to understand that we live in a world of intense energies; energies emitted not just from your smart phone, digital television, computer, or game console, but also from the ever-increasing number of microwave cell towers, power stations, and other electromagnetic field (EMF) emitters.

The average person spends over five hours a day in front of a computer screen. These types of EMF exposures can quickly and easily disrupt your own very sensitive energy fields. More importantly they can fry your nervous system and over-stimulate your organs, including your brain, and that can easily induce insomnia in anyone, and most often in ultra-sensitive individuals just like you. As with any other disruptors, energy or EMF over-stimulation can complicate the insomnia dilemma by also directly disrupting your sensitive hormone balance.

GOT GHOSTS?

Okay, for those who are easily spooked or who don't believe in such things as ghosts, let's just refer to these unseen forces as "energy attachments". There is much to be said about ghosts, hauntings, and ghost busting, most of which we will not get into within the scope of this book. But if *you* have an interest in ghosts and how they affect you and your loved ones, do a little hunting of your own. There is plenty of this material out there either on television, on the web, or in your favorite ghost hunting book. In fact, ghost hunting has become a hot commodity lately with sales of electronic ghost regalia on the rise world-wide. I myself find the whole genre quite fascinating, and the exploration of ghost phenomenon is one of my favorite endeavors outside of my healing practice.

What you will learn about ghosts when you look past all the Hollywood glam is that no matter what we call them, these discarnate energies do exist, they are real, and they can affect us physically and emotionally. If they become attached to your energy field or reside in any area of your business or home, particularly in your sleeping area, like other EMF emitters, these energy attachments can lead to insomnia, especially in ultra-sensitive individuals. How does this happen? Simple. Ghosts are made of energy. *We* are made of energy. When these energies intermingle it can affect us in profound and unsuspecting ways, and can most certainly keep us awake. In fact, a good majority of individuals who experience insomnia are indeed being affected in one way or another by these energy attachments, often without a clue as to what's transpiring.

For those who have not experienced the effects of unseen energies, it may be hard to comprehend how they could affect your sleep, your dreams, and truly the quality of your life. For the many that have experienced spirit activity, such as my wife and I, you can be sure that unwanted or even *wanted* energy attachments can wreak havoc on your sleep. If you feel that you or your loved ones are not the only ones occupying your sleeping room, I strongly encourage you to get a clearing from a proven energy worker or ghost buster, someone who has a track record of clearing energies.

In the meanwhile, you can take some practical measures on your own. Before you lay down to go to sleep command these energy attachments to leave your space at once. Be firm, be consistent, and perseverant. If at first it seems they are not heeding your request, raise your energy and your intent to a higher frequency. If after several weeks of nightly requests, after reciting your energy clearing mantras, and after a smoke or smudge ceremony, you still feel their presence, do seek out a real life ghost buster. They're out there.

Spirit activity in sleeping rooms is a reality and a very real sleep disruptor. Please take this seriously. If you need further guidance on this subject please contact my office.

HORMONAL INSOMNIA

EMF emitters and ghosts are by no means the only unseen triggers that can cause insomnia. Low progesterone levels from any cause and for any reason, and *especially* after a hysterectomy, can result in sleep problems, not just falling asleep but staying asleep, as well. If you've had a hysterectomy, or have reached those menopausal years, or have low progesterone levels for any other reason, supplementation with topical progesterone can help restore that quality sleep your body and mind are craving.

MARSHA is a sixty-something woman endowed with a knack for spirituality. She had worked all her life to hone her spiritual gifts, studying Hinduism, Buddhism, and the like, and partaking and even teaching yoga and spirituality to other gifted individuals. An excellent homemaker and a very generous and giving woman, Marsha directed much of her physical and emotional energy and attention to her loving husband and to her very needy and very co-dependent 28-year old son.

Not unlike herself, her ultra-sensitive son had a very difficult time adapting to the stressors of everyday life. Like many sensitive individuals he struggled with his identity and purpose on this planet, and he'd grown into quite an introvert. He had a difficult time holding down a traditional job and his resultant poverty state necessitated that he tap into the financial and emotional bank from his parents, especially Marsha, who was clearly connected to her son in a special way. These two clearly had some serious karma to work through.

Being the sensitive, generous, and compassionate person that she was, Marsha too often gave into her needy son, giving substantial amounts of money, worrying about his health, making sure he was eating properly; she provided for his every need. This went on for over a decade. But all that giving, without receiving any emotional support in return, took a toll on Marsha's physical and emotional health. She began to develop cysts on her breasts and her ovaries, one of the most common outcomes from this type of long-term behavior.

Unfortunately, rather than working to reduce cystic growth by reducing estrogen levels, her traditional medical practitioners deemed that Marsha required surgical intervention. A hysterectomy was performed. That was followed by a lumpectomy which was followed by reconstructive breast surgery; more than enough PTSD for anyone, especially a sensitive one. Within three months following the hysterectomy Marsha found herself in my office complaining of chronic insomnia. She had tried all the usual prescription medicines with poor results, and was now willing to do anything to get sleep. I knew exactly what was needed to make that happen, progesterone supplementation. We immediately began a high dose topical progesterone regimen to replenish Marsha's dwindling progesterone stores, dwindling because the primary progesterone-producing organs had been removed in the hysterectomy. I also included several estrogen-lowering supplements to balance the high estrogen levels behind her cystic dilemma.

Within six weeks Marsha's sleep began to improve significantly, from a mere three to four hours a night to seven to eight hours nightly. During the transition period, we did also employ several natural sleep remedies that included valerian, skullcap, and melatonin, but her need for these products diminished as her progesterone levels began to balance.

After catching up on months of sleep deprivation, Marsha exclaimed that she felt like a new person, once again able to enjoy her spiritual studies. That was when I decided to have an in-depth discussion with her about her over-nurturing behavior. It took a few emotional clearing sessions and several past-life regressions but Marsha finally understood the health implications of her over-nurturing; she finally got the message loud and clear. She ultimately made peace with her son and the lessons that were his, and their karmic connection, and she went on to become a powerful and respected spiritual teacher, something she had been aspiring to all of her life.

SLEEP ON IT

But not too long. If you are a female suffering from chronic sleep deprivation, it's time to examine all the insomnia triggers in your life, especially low progesterone levels. Progesterone and estrogen imbalances aren't the only culprit behind your sleep challenges, but if they're out of balance for any reason they are definitely part of the problem. The solution? Get your hormones checked and balanced by a qualified holistic practitioner. And while you're there, open a dialogue to investigate all of the *other* sleep disruptors that have likely been hiding in plain sight for some time. You can learn all you need to know about these disruptors and how to clear them naturally in my book "You Are Sensitive!"

HORMONE TRUTH:

Sleep deprivation is detrimental to your health. Progesterone levels should be checked and balanced through applied kinesiology before starting on any other sleep remedies.

HORMONE BALANCING REGIMEN FOR INSOMNIA

1. Progesterone cream

<u>For women still cycling:</u>

Topical progesterone cream ¼ to ½ teaspoonfuls rubbed into breast, stomach, thighs, or inner arm once daily at bedtime on your cycle days 12 through 26. The first day of your cycle is the first day of bleeding.

<u>For women no longer cycling:</u>

Topical progesterone cream ¼ to ½ teaspoonfuls rubbed into breast, stomach, thighs, or inner arm once daily at bedtime on calendar days 1 through 25 only.

- Rotate application site every two to three days
- It may take two to three months or longer to notice full improvement of symptoms, so be patient
- Hormone levels should be checked through applied kinesiology throughout the balancing period at approximately three to four week intervals

2. Inositol 500 to 1000mg orally one-half hour before bedtime as needed for sleep

- Inositol is not addictive and may be used on a continuous basis indefinitely
- Inositol has no significant interactions with any prescription medicines

Fibrocystic Breasts and Ovaries

HIGH ESTROGEN CAN LEAD TO CYSTIC GROWTH

How many women do you know that have reported painful and uncomfortable fibroid cysts in their breasts or ovaries? Here's one for the record books. In my healing practice literally *95 percent* of all the women I work with have reported feeling pain from cysts on their breasts or ovaries or both. It's an enormous problem that no one seems to be paying attention to.

Tens of millions of women are racing through their daily activities while fibroid cysts continue to grow larger and larger. Why is that? That's because these tens of millions of women have no idea that they have high estrogen levels. That's right. And high estrogen levels drive cystic growth anywhere and everywhere. We are in the midst of the **high estrogen crisis**, and unwittingly you may very well be a club member.

Yes, the media has poked fun at women in menopause, blaming the stereotypical emotional tirades, edginess, and moodiness on *low* estrogen levels. The fact is, just the opposite is true. Most women have *high* estrogen levels and they don't have a clue. What's more, the health practitioners caring for these menopausal women are *giving estrogen* to treat menopausal symptoms and in the process are exacerbating cystic growth everywhere in the body.

If you're a female between the ages of puberty and sixty-five, there's a good chance you have fibroid cysts growing in your body right now, and you probably don't even know it.

SIGNS AND SYMPTOMS OF FIBROID CYSTS

- Back pain
- Pelvic pain, around your period or any time
- Tender or painful breasts, around your period or any time
- Painful, heavy, or difficult periods, often with clotting
- Unexplained cystic growth on any area or organ of the body

HORMONAL GROWTH SPURT

So why is fibroid cystic growth so rampant on this planet? That's because estrogen levels are on the rise globally, for a variety of reasons discussed earlier. But no matter the reason or the cause, it is imperative that *every* woman understand that the high estrogen crisis is directly responsible for the explosive incidence of fibrocystic disease. Even more important and more disturbing is the fact that unbridled high estrogen levels can lead to serious health consequences, up to and including endometriosis, and breast, uterine, or ovarian cancer. Without a doubt high estrogen can have catastrophic effects on the quality and duration of your life span. Hence, it's imperative that you have a full grasp on what may be lurking inside you as you read this material.

Here's a snapshot of the hormone profile in women who suffer from fibrocystic disease:

LOW progesterone plus HIGH estrogen = FIBROID CYSTS

COMMONLY OVERLOOKED CAUSES OF FIBROCYSTIC BREASTS AND OVARIES

- Post traumatic stress disorder (PTSD) from rape, war, violence, accidents
- Over-nurturing others while under-nurturing self
- Stressful lifestyle
- Hysterectomy
- Birth control pills or devices
- Harsh words
- Negative thinking
- Prescription estrogen medicines
- Iodine deficiency
- Unhealthy relationships
- Lack of sexual expression
- Genetics
- Anger, resentment, guilt, shame, or any negative emotion
- Pesticides and chemical byproducts
- **High estrogen levels**

HYSTERECTOMY - THE VICIOUS HORMONAL CYCLE

High estrogen levels can be produced over time from a variety of factors. Yet, no matter how they become elevated the result is always the same, the ultimate destruction of the reproductive organs. That's why we are seeing so many cases of endometriosis, breast cysts, ovarian cysts, and a meteoric rise in hormonal cancers. The medical community has responded to this epidemic by offering to remove the damaged tissue rather than correct the underlying problem caused by high estrogen. It's called a hysterectomy.

This is a travesty; a travesty because hundreds of thousands of unnecessary hysterectomies are performed each year that could have been avoided had gynecologists and other practitioners paid closer attention to the whole clinical picture of their female patients. Instead, most of these practitioners responded to these estrogenically-induced symptoms by removing precious reproductive tissue, a knee-jerk reaction that is unfortunately a standard of practice in the traditional medical community.

DO IT YOURSELF

But it's not too late to affect a positive change on your own and help avoid the knife and other unhealthy consequences. Believe it or not, you can easily and quickly reverse the rise of estrogen levels and halt the cystic growth that is likely occurring within you even as you read this material. It's something you can do in the privacy of your own home whenever you choose and as often as you choose, and it's something you have complete control over. It requires no drugs and no surgeries and doesn't require a co-pay. But there is one catch. You must be willing to be honest with yourself when you come face to face with it. And you *must* come face to face with it. What is this powerful and magical hormonal healer? Nurture.

How does it work? You take more, they take less. By that of course I mean you must nurture yourself more and nurture all the others — husbands, lovers, boyfriends, children, bosses, friends, *less*. That doesn't mean you don't love them or care about them. Of course you do. When you explain to them that you're making this behavioral change to potentially save your own life, they'll understand. What *you* need to understand is this:

**Over-nurturing others while under-nurturing yourself
leads to high estrogen levels.**

Yes, there exists a very real biochemical cascade of events that occurs over time that will faithfully follow this equation. It may take several years, even several decades to show up but if you continue to give to others while depriving yourself of nurturing, both physically and emotionally, your estrogen levels *will* begin to rise. It's that simple. And it's important to note that this over-nurturing behavior can begin as early as birth, and most definitely by puberty, and for most women seems to never let up, ever — unless and until they recognize and correct this pervasive female gender miscue. The solution? Start taking care of yourself first.

AVOID THE HORSE URINE

From my perspective, no prescription medicine has taken a greater toll on the health and wellbeing of the menopausal woman as the prescription substance known as the conjugated estrogens, a mixture of estrogen hormones, which remarkably are still in use today.

Released in 1942, the innovator brand of conjugated estrogens was coined from the source of its parent compound **pre**gnant **mar**e urine, or female horse urine. This theoretically naturally-derived product is made up of conjugated estrogens, and over its 71-year history has been the source of more hormonal disruptions worldwide than any other prescription hormonal remedy. That's because at the end of the day prescription medicines that contain conjugated estrogens are nothing short of potent estrogen, a compound that is largely responsible for instigating and perpetuating the global high estrogen crisis.

Thirty billion doses later, this prescription estrogenic product has become world famous and a hugely profitable blockbuster drug because of its ability to squelch hot flashes, the key complaint plaguing menopausal women. But what many women and most traditional practitioners don't realize is that having hot flashes, which is generally indicative of *low* estrogen levels, is preferable to having *high* estrogen, a dangerous and precarious hormonal state of imbalance.

HIGH OR LOW: YOU ROLL THE DICE

The truth is, having hot flashes is a blessing in disguise. Why a blessing? They can be miserable, and keep you awake at night, and soak your clothes. What's so blessed about that? The blessing is that if you have hot flashes you likely have *low* estrogen and are far less likely to be bothered by fibrocystic breasts or ovaries, or cystic growth of any kind, and far less likely to develop hormonal cancers. The bad news is that despite what mainstream medicine may believe, far fewer women suffer from hot flashes than suffer from fibrocystic tissue growth issues. Which do you choose? Hot flashes or the real potential for developing cysts and hormonal cancers? You roll the dice.

Not sure what's going on inside you? You're not alone. Millions of women along with their practitioners don't seem to know either. If you believe you have fibroid cysts in your breast, or any lump in your breast, or if you have unexplained back or pelvic pain, or heavy bleeding around your period, even if you're no longer cycling, get your hormones checked by a qualified practitioner promptly so that high estrogen levels can be properly balanced.

CARRIE arrived in my office in great pain. A 48-year old practicing Buddhist, she had been suffering from focalized pelvic pain and generalized back pain for several years. Carrie explained that these symptoms seemed to be far worse around her period, but her period was so irregular she hadn't actually bled in three months. When she did, the flow was heavy and full of clots. Gynecological evaluations, x-rays, and Pap smears revealed no abnormalities. Even blood tests for progesterone and estrogen hormones ordered by her gynecologist were unremarkable. What was remarkable was that Carrie was in obvious physical distress.

During the course of taking her medical history, Carrie confessed that she'd had difficult and irregular periods most of her adult life, and that it wasn't unusual for her flow to be painful and clotty. She'd also had ongoing issues with fibrocystic lumps which she palpated while performing her monthly breast self-checks. Her gynecologist concurred that the cysts were likely benign, but at the same time she prescribed estradiol, potent estrogen, to manage the occasional hot flashes that Carrie had begun to experience.

Carrie also made mention that her mother had endured similar issues during her hormonal evolution. She too had experienced painful periods, cystic breasts, and pelvic pain, which led Carrie to believe that she herself might just have to endure the same fate as her mother. Sit and suffer. I couldn't disagree more, and assured Carrie that we don't always have to fall victim to family genetics. I explained that her estrogen levels were high and have likely been high most of her adult life, partly due to genetics, partly due to her continuous over-nurturing and coddling of her high maintenance mother. Unfortunately, the addition of the prescription estradiol was making matters worse by pushing estrogen levels over the edge, which in turn encouraged the growth of her cystic tissue.

We began by immediately stopping the estradiol, and then added topical progesterone cream ½ teaspoonful nightly on the calendar days one through twenty-five of each month. This would help alleviate the hot flashes while bringing back to balance the all-important progesterone/estrogen ratio. Nattokinase, a natural fibrinolytic agent, along with several other estrogen modulating products were started per my instructions to help slowly begin breaking down the cysts. And they did their job faithfully.

Carrie was wonderfully compliant and continued the regimen as I directed. It took a good six months or so but her cysts and the pain they caused began to diminish noticeably. Those elevated estrogen levels not only began to fall, but Carrie also began to allow her mother to work through her own lessons, hence liberating Carrie from much of the guilt she had been carrying for so many years. This potent nutritional and emotional combination did the trick, as it often does. Allowing her mother to take more responsibility for herself was a wonderful relief for Carrie, but also a powerful lesson in disguise for her mother, who surprisingly enjoyed *her* new independence, thank you very much.

A year later Carrie reported that she was feeling better than ever, with only a rare hot flash and no further breast or pelvic pain concerns. Carrie had successfully managed to balance those high circulating estrogen levels and continues to get them checked holistically at least once yearly.

IGNORANCE TRULY IS BLISS... AND SOMETIMES DANGEROUS

As we've seen, high estrogen levels can create unhealthy and even dangerous cellular changes in susceptible and sensitive individuals, but if you're not paying careful attention you may miss the high estrogen warning lights altogether. Yes, difficult periods and fibroid cysts are often the first signs that your estrogen is too high, but cystic growth on *any* organ and *any* other place on the body can also be a sign that estrogen is revving too high. Although poorly documented and even more poorly diagnosed, cystic growth on non-reproductive organs can also be the result of high circulating estrogen. And in fact, I have had the privilege of observing a number of such occurrences in my years of practice.

SALLY is a 48-year old woman that I have known for many years. Sensitive, misunderstood, and very much a hypochondriac, Sally settled down with her sensitive husband and the family retriever in a small town in California. I had lost touch with her over the years, but we finally did reconnect by telephone in early 2004.

We caught up on the chit chat and all the usual salutations were exchanged. Then we came to that fateful moment. Sally knew what I did for a living and seemingly out of nowhere she began to regurgitate all of her health dilemmas, which I must admit caught me by surprise. I had no intention whatsoever of delving into this woman's convoluted health matters and as a rule avoid working with family and friends at all costs, for reasons that I won't expound on here. Nevertheless, this innocent phone call reeled me into a situation I could not free myself from. I took a deep breath...

Sally went on to explain at length and in explicit detail all of the hormonal issues that had beset her over the past 15 years. She had been diagnosed with fibrocystic breasts, complained of unexplained pelvic pain, and suffered with irregular cycles for the past 10 years. Then she laid down the bombshell. She explained with tears in her eyes that she had been experiencing upper right quadrant pain and discomfort for almost five years, and had also been losing weight during that period of time. She was clearly distraught about the potential of what this could be, and frankly I too was a bit concerned. This was not a good combination of symptoms.

As much as I didn't want to get into this with Sally, I was already in, hook, line, and sinker; the plight and pitfall of my overly compassionate nature. She had been down the traditional route with blood tests, ultrasounds, and physical exams, yet these revealed nothing conclusive. Her doctors told her it was all in her head. Yes, there could have been some of that in this case, but I just felt they were overlooking something, and if for no other reason than to calm her fears, I was determined to find it. Working long distance by phone, I performed a full intuitive and energetic workup *my* way.

We uncovered several key organ imbalances that traditional methods had missed. Sally had a gallbladder full of stones, her liver energy was checking out of balance, and she had a hormone profile consistent with PCOS, Polycystic Ovary Syndrome, which included very high estrogen levels. Sally was relieved to learn that there was some non-life threatening explanations for all these nagging symptoms, and so was I. We began a PCOS regimen to balance her hormones, and added several additional supplements for liver support. I also asked her to perform a gallbladder flush per our protocol, which she immediately did. To Sally's great surprise her gallbladder flush produced over 100 gallstones which were impacted in the gallbladder, the symptoms of which often include right upper quadrant discomfort.

Over the next eight months most of Sally's symptoms diminished noticeably and her "liver" pain had begun to improve, but never fully subsided. Instead it waxed and waned, and continued to be a source of much turmoil and emotional worry, given Sally's hypochondriac nature. Her allopathic doctors were satisfied with her symptomatic improvement and were not motivated to further workup her pain and weight loss. Yet I still felt there was something else at play, something everyone else was missing: liver cysts.

Sally was finally able to get one of her doctors to repeat the ultrasound to take a closer second look, and there it was. Sally had developed a fibrocystic growth on her liver and another small cyst on her lung. Her life-long undiagnosed high estrogen levels combined with her extremely over-nurturing nature had over the years resulted in cysts growing on her liver and lung. Sally was once again relieved to learn that the source or her "mysterious" symptoms were relatively innocuous cystic growths; growths that could be managed naturally using the proper holistic protocol.

I enhanced her estrogen balancing regimen and advised her to stay on this regimen for at least several years, and she has. Sally continues that regimen faithfully to this day. Her liver pain remains greatly diminished, and after several lengthy counseling sessions I was able to make her understand how her sensitive, over-nurturing, and emotional nature was at the root cause of these symptoms. Yes, there were more tears, but they weren't tears of fear. They were tears of gratefulness. I believe she finally got the message.

Today, Sally is a well-adjusted, emotionally balanced woman and lives her life with more calm and content than ever before. These days our phone conversations are filled only with positivity, and conversation about fond memories of years gone by.

HORMONE TRUTH:

If you've been over-nurturing others and under-nurturing yourself for too long you likely have high estrogen levels, despite what any blood test might reveal. And that will put you at risk for developing cysts anywhere in or on your body

HORMONE BALANCING REGIMEN FOR FIBROCYSTIC BREASTS AND OVARIES

1. Progesterone cream

For women still cycling:

Topical progesterone cream ¼ to ½ teaspoonfuls rubbed into breast, stomach, thighs, or inner arm once daily at bedtime on your cycle days 12 through 26. The first day of your cycle is the first day of bleeding.

For women no longer cycling:

Topical progesterone cream ¼ to ½ teaspoonfuls rubbed into breast, stomach, thighs, or inner arm once daily at bedtime on calendar days 1 through 25 only.

- Rotate application site every two to three days
- It may take two to three months or longer to notice full improvement of symptoms, so be patient
- Hormone levels should be checked through applied kinesiology throughout the balancing period at approximately three to four week intervals

2. DIM (diindolylmethane) once to twice daily or as directed on bottle continuously until estrogen levels are balanced

- Do not take if you become pregnant or are lactating
- Estrogen levels should be checked through applied kinesiology throughout the balancing period at approximately three to four week intervals

3. Nattokinase 100mg once to twice daily with food

- If you are taking prescription blood thinners or blood pressure medicines, or have a history of bleeding tendency, get professional guidance before you start
- It may take several months or longer to break down cystic tissue, so be patient

4. Flax lignan capsules 2 to 6 capsules daily with food in divided doses.

- Take each dose with a large glass of water
- It may take several months or longer to break down cystic tissue, so be patient

Weight Gain

LOW PROGESTERONE CAN LEAD TO WEIGHT GAIN

Saying that weight gain is a concern on the minds of most women would be a gross understatement for the ages. Weight control and figure management seems to be one of the most pervasive thought patterns among women of all ages, everywhere. Concerns about weight and body shape drive millions of women and men to buy basketfuls of diet pills; purchase unspoken quantities of gym memberships and portioned "diet" foods, and creates more self-esteem damage than one can possibly imagine. These desperate individuals spend the better part of 50 *billion* dollars annually on weight loss efforts. The truth is most individuals will spend whatever it takes on literally everything imaginable in an attempt to lose weight and "look good".

It simply amazes me then how so many millions of individuals who desperately want to lose weight and look trim fail to understand the role that hormone balance plays in this all-important arena of vanity, self-esteem, and self-worth.

GET THE PICTURE

Here's something you must begin to understand if you truly want to be healthy and become your perfect weight and size. It starts with having a realistic expectation about how you're really supposed to look.

The fact is each of us has an image in our minds about how we wish to physically appear to others; yet unless you are metabolically "wired", genetically coded to be thin, forcing yourself to become thin is not healthy in any way. Not everybody is supposed to be skinny. Unfortunately in this society a vast majority of women have a skewed vision about how they are supposed to look based on social pressures, on how their peers look, and of course on what they see on TV and in magazines.

And then of course it behooves us to accurately define the term "skinny". Skinny to one woman may mean fat to another, and vice versa. It's all about preconceived notions about how we appear to ourselves and to others and the societal programming we've been exposed to. But let's be real. Much of this programming has been grossly exaggerated by unhealthy, and in many cases, truly unflattering role models. Many of these role models, celebrities and the like, are truly hormonal and emotional messes themselves, often living unhealthy lifestyles, and consuming the nutritional input of a stapler. Please, honestly ask yourself this question: is this the person I wish to become, really?

WORK IT

It's also important to understand that many men and women are working too hard to force their metabolism to fit a skeletal structure that wasn't designed to handle that weight. In other words, some people really do have big bones and were built and wired to weigh more than other people. Others are built to weigh less. Artificially forcing your metabolism to achieve a weight or image you have in mind may not be what your physiology, your metabolism, or your genetics can accomplish without creating new health problems. The result of "trying too hard" can actually *create* hormonal imbalances, among other health issues. And you really don't want that. So stop working so hard to become a weight and size that may not be metabolically appropriate for you, and set realistic expectations based on the size and shape you were *meant to be*.

How do you know what weight or shape you were genetically destined to be? It's simple. Start by balancing your hormones. Once they are properly balanced and you begin eating foods appropriate to your metabolic type, in time you will *automatically* fall into your proper weight and shape. That's how the body was designed to work.

COMMONLY OVERLOOKED CAUSES OF WEIGHT GAIN

- Unresolved emotional hurt (often associated with anorexia nervosa and/or bulimia)
- Genetics
- Depression (which can ensue due to unresolved emotional hurt)
- Poor diet choices
- Large portion sizes
- Hysterectomy

- Candidiasis, Candida yeast infection
- Lack of regular exercise
- Prescription medications
- Thyroid imbalances
- Iodine deficiency
- **Low progesterone**

AVERT THE HURT

As you can see, a number of lifestyle miscues play a role in the weight gain dilemma. One miscue that deserves your undivided attention and is almost always overlooked by health practitioners is the issue of **unresolved emotional hurt**. Every one of us has experienced our share of being hurt emotionally and often physically at least to some degree, often damaging our confidence and self-esteem, especially in women. Unless these traumas are resolved through emotional clearing techniques or holistic-based counseling, they can frequently result in eating disorders, up to and including anorexia nervosa or bulimia. If you have food issues, food guilt, or any other unhealthy approach to eating, it is imperative that these be cleared and resolved in order to achieve any long-lasting weight management.

I'm not going to cover this important concept in this book, but there are many other resources out there that do cover it in great detail. I also encourage you to read my book "You Are Sensitive!" for a deeper look at how to address emotional hurt that may be causing your weight gain. But do know this. Unresolved emotional hurt will ultimately lead to low progesterone and high estrogen, and as you will see, low progesterone levels play a pivotal role in the weight management picture.

IT'S ALL ABOUT YOUR METABOLISM

If you are serious about losing weight, it is absolutely crucial for you to understand this very simple, yet very important fact. Your thyroid function, which is your key metabolic organ, ultimately controls your weight balance. If you fail to correct and balance your thyroid function, you WILL NOT lose weight, unless you artificially accelerate your metabolism through stimulant pills or over-exercise. Any weight loss accomplished using these methods alone will not last. Sound familiar? Perhaps you've been there before. You can exercise 24 hours a day and you can eat like a canary. But if you do not correct thyroid function you will never fully achieve your weight goals. In the end, the original weight will eventually come back, and then some, just for good measure. Regardless of all those weight loss products and weight program pitches you see on television at the beginning of each new year, if you want to lose weight through the process nature intended and *keep it off*, you must correct the underlying cause: poor thyroid function.

FIX ME, PLEASE!

So how do you get your thyroid in perfect balance, the way your genetics intended? It starts by addressing two key areas in your body:

Low progesterone levels
Low iodine levels

Let's focus on low progesterone levels, the more common of the two imbalances. Not to underplay the prevalence and importance of correcting low iodine stores, it's very important and it's pretty darn common. We'll talk about correcting low iodine levels in another chapter. But for now, let's be clear about this: The most effective and most important thing you can do to lose weight and keep it off is to correct low progesterone levels.

What does your progesterone level have to do with your weight? Here's the simplified explanation. Progesterone must be at optimum levels for the thyroid to make and utilize what we call T3, the active thyroid hormone. Low progesterone levels mean less T3 is being made, which means that thyroid function will suffer. When thyroid function is low, your metabolism is low. The result over time is weight gain.

Low progesterone levels over time will lead to
low thyroid function
Low thyroid function over time will lead to weight gain

It's really that simple. Sure, we could over-analyze this concept until nausea sets in, but at the end of the day we'll still come up with the same conclusion. Most women on this planet have low progesterone levels. If you're a woman who has reached the age of puberty, there's a very good chance *you* have low progesterone levels. It matters not if you are 13, 30 or 80. If you have not balanced your progesterone levels and addressed other lifestyle miscues such as eating properly, exercising, and processing emotional hurt, you could very well be experiencing weight gain you do *not* want.

TAKE A PILL

Hormonal disruptors are everywhere in our environment, yet nearly every one of these disruptors can be avoided or averted if one is paying close attention. Most certainly one disruptor we have the choice of avoiding altogether is hormonal birth control.

Let me be clear. Although a hot box topic these days, I am not against using birth control. I am merely pointing out that birth control pills and devices containing estrogenic ingredients can slowly, insidiously, and without your knowledge or permission, disrupt your delicate reproductive hormone profile. Depending on the type of pill used, hormone birth control can cause an unhealthy and sometimes unpredictable lowering of progesterone and force estrogen levels to climb in unnatural ways. The result of this shift often results in weight gain, among other serious adverse effects, and these types of hormonal disruptions are particularly troublesome in sensitive individuals, like you.

BARBARA scheduled an appointment with me to address her sudden weight gain. A 42-year old corporate executive, she had gained over 40 pounds over the last three years, and the weight just kept on climbing, weighing in at 167 pounds at our first visit in a five-foot-four frame. Clearly frustrated, she had done everything she could think of to stay trim, but nothing seemed to work. It's as though her weight had a mind of its own. Barbara exercised regularly, in fact her workouts were almost too much by my standard; 90-minute cardio training plus an hour or more of weight training five days a week. Her diet was mostly on target with sensible protein intake and a balanced variety of vegetables and grains. Despite all of this, Barbara could not seem to halt the weight progression.

I checked Barbara's hormone profile through kinesiology and discovered what I almost always discover in these types of situations. Barbara's progesterone levels were very low, and her thyroid function was correspondingly low. She was metabolically deficient due to low progesterone levels. Now we just needed to determine how this progesterone deficiency came about. Before I could utter another word, Barbara confessed that her job had become exceptionally stressful over the past three years, especially after her promotion to division manager. She had also just recently stopped using her oral birth control pill, which she had been taking for over 20 years.

As is often the case, the use of long term hormonal birth control had "confused" her hormonal system, creating a typical distortion of the hormone profile: low progesterone and high estrogen. The low progesterone levels over time had resulted in low thyroid function. To complicate things even further her family doctor had prescribed the thyroid stimulant levothyroxine, to combat the weight gain. Unfortunately, as is always the case, levothyroxine failed to address the underlying thyroid problem, low progesterone levels, and the weight gain continued unabated.

I asked Barbara to taper off the levothyroxine over a four-week period to avoid any rebound fatigue. I also started her on a topical progesterone cream regimen to raise her progesterone levels. She was quite compliant and quite surprised *and pleased* to find that within three weeks of starting this regimen she had lost five pounds. Walking 40 minutes daily and eating her sensible balanced diet, Barbara's weight continued to drop off at a healthy pace, about one pound every week. She continued on this regimen faithfully and during this process made another healthy resolution, leaving her high pressure job in lieu of something more attuned to her energy: counseling teens on the merits of self-esteem and proper nutrition. A perfect fit.

By sticking with her healthy habits, Barbara has been able to maintain her new weight of 128 pounds ever since and is more delighted than ever to achieve this life-long weight target.

IDEAL WEIGHT IS WITHIN REACH

Your goal of a perfect shape and a perfect weight is most definitely within reach and most certainly achievable. And it starts by getting yourself hormonally balanced. Add a dose of sensible nutrition, healthy thinking, and start paying attention to that emotional chatter that needs to be processed and cleared, and you too can accomplish the weight and shape nature intended for you. Please do set realistic expectations and time frames for the process, and when you do, you too will delight in feeling confident and comfortable in your body once again. Need help? Reach out to a qualified holistic practitioner who has experience in hormone balancing. They'll get you on the path to success.

HORMONE TRUTH:

If you've been struggling with your weight for years, no weight plan or diet pill will keep the weight off until you balance your progesterone levels. Clearing emotional sludge will help your progesterone levels and your weight stay balanced.

HORMONE BALANCING REGIMEN FOR WEIGHT GAIN

1. Progesterone cream

For women still cycling:

Topical progesterone cream ¼ to ½ teaspoonfuls rubbed into breast, stomach, thighs, or inner arm once daily at bedtime on your cycle days 12 through 26. The first day of your cycle is the first day of bleeding.

For women no longer cycling:

Topical progesterone cream ¼ to ½ teaspoonfuls rubbed into breast, stomach, thighs, or inner arm once daily at bedtime on calendar days 1 through 25 only.

- Rotate application site every two to three days
- It may take two to three months or longer to notice full improvement of symptoms, so be patient
- Hormone levels should be checked through applied kinesiology throughout the balancing period at approximately three to four week intervals

2. Iodine 150 to 300mcg once daily in the morning at least ½ hour before food.

- Higher doses may be required in some cases. Do not exceed the above doses without professional guidance
- Although true iodine allergies are quite rare, do not take supplemental iodine without guidance if you have a documented allergy to iodine
- Iodine levels should be checked through applied kinesiology throughout the balancing period at approximately three to four week intervals

Low Libido

LOW PROGESTERONE CAN LEAD TO LOW LIBIDO

Here's a topic hot on the minds of everyone everywhere, right? One would think so, yet millions of individuals worldwide suffer silently with low or non-existent sex drive, never discussing this matter with anyone. Not only are these individuals not interested in having sex, many have completely forgotten what it is like to have a lively libido. It's been gone so long they have simply learned to live without one. Is this you?

The truth is, an unfortunate majority of women, as well as plenty of men, have actually forsaken the notion of sexual activity altogether. Their "mojo" is gone. Not just on lunch break, but completely left the building. What's going on here? For most women the answer is low progesterone levels.

Yes, you've heard it before. Low progesterone levels can wreak all kinds of havoc on the human body and spirit. It can also leave us sexually listless. There are a number of environmental issues you may have not considered that can lead to low libido, and each of these will ultimately result in the same common denominator. Progesterone stores are compromised. Restore yours and you too can bring back that lovin' feeling.

COMMONLY OVERLOOKED CAUSES OF LOW LIBIDO

- Post traumatic stress disorder (PTSD) from rape, war, violence, accidents
- Over-nurturing others while under-nurturing self
- Birth control pills or devices
- Negative thinking
- Unhealthy relationships
- Genetics
- Anger, resentment, guilt, shame, or any negative emotion
- Sexual trauma
- Antidepressant medications
- Hypertension medications

- Hysterectomy
- Postpartum Depression
- Lifestyle stressors or hectic schedule
- Poor nutrition
- **Low progesterone**

As expected, there is a variety of culprits that can steal away your libido, slowly, insidiously and without your permission. Most of these lifestyle factors are typically overlooked and become disguised within the routines of your life, so much so that you may not even realize your libido has gone away. Let's take a closer look at several key libido saboteurs.

MENOPAUSE AND ANDROPAUSE: THE GREAT HORMONAL SHIFTS

The life shift we know as menopause, or the male counterpart I refer to as andropause, are powerful periods of time in our lives when hormones shift, our perspective about life shifts, and our understanding about our place in that life also shifts. It's also a time when your libido is subject to change, and most always in a less-desirable direction.

Along with weight gain, insomnia, anxiety, and fatigue, low libido is one of the hallmark signs that you've entered that magical cycle of life we are all going to go through at some point in time, the "pause". And like it or not, your hormones are responsible. For women, fading progesterone levels are the primary hormonal culprit. For men, it's typically a shift in the progesterone to estrogen ratios and sagging testosterone levels that are responsible. We'll discuss the nuances of male menopause in the Andropause chapter.

Oh, sure there are other nutritional factors that contribute to a lackluster libido, but for the female gender you can bet low progesterone is part of your libido betrayal. But all is not lost. Women, if your libido is faltering, supplementing with topical progesterone cream during this 5 to 15-year life cycle can help restore your youthful prowess. Feeling sexually listless? Reach out to a qualified holistic practitioner. They can evaluate your hormone status and help put you and your libido in a happier place. And happy is good.

But out there lurks yet another commonly-overlooked libido destroyer; a libido predator so insidious and so prevalent, you may not realize what hit you. The fact is, if you are one of the over 30 million Americans using prescription antidepressants to manage your low mood, you may be sabotaging your libido without realizing it.

GOOD MOOD OR SEX DRIVE?

You may have to choose, especially if you're taking prescription medicines for symptoms of depression. That's because prescription antidepressants like fluoxetine, paroxetine, sertraline, citalopram, and others like them, are notorious for disrupting a normal libido and for causing sexual performance issues. How do they accomplish this? Forcing serotonin and other brain chemical levels to rise through artificial means can distort their normal biological activity and negatively affect your libido.

Not only that, selective serotonin reuptake inhibitors or SSRI's like fluoxetine, paroxetine, and citalopram can actually cause progesterone levels to fall, and that can ironically hamper the improvement of mood we are wishing to accomplish. Although the mechanism is not fully understood or recognized by science, over the years I have indeed observed that individuals taking SSRI type antidepressants often have lower progesterone levels than their clinical picture would dictate. As a matter of record I have also noted that the reverse is also true; that women with low progesterone levels have low measurable serotonin levels, substantiating the finding that low progesterone often leads to low mood. That doesn't bode well for women in menopause who routinely have low progesterone, and not surprisingly, more mood issues overall.

How about the happy medium? How about a good mood *and* a healthy sex life? You *can* have both. It starts by getting your progesterone levels balanced *before* you commit to taking a prescription antidepressant medication. Once you become hormonally and nutritionally balanced, mood issues often slowly fade away, and often while you're not paying attention.

Please be clear. I am not suggesting that you stop your prescription antidepressants. These medicines should never be stopped suddenly or without guidance from a health professional. But I am suggesting this. At the end of the day you don't have to choose between mood and libido. Simply choose to discuss this matter with a holistic health practitioner you trust. They can help get you on the happy track naturally.

AMANDA is an emotionally-inert 59-year old woman who originally came to see me about her fibrocystic tissue growth in her ovaries and breasts. She reported back pain, pelvic pain, and lower abdominal cramping which seemed to wax and wane around her period, and so did her mood. Amanda had been through the typical battery of tests: blood draws, multiple ultra-sounds, several CAT scans, yet her gynecologist could not find a cause for the cystic growth.

Before I could even give her my impression of her hormone miscues, Amanda leaned into me, lowered her voice and spelled out the *real* reason for her visit with me. Without flinching, Amanda confided that she'd completely lost interest in sex, and that she was afraid that her husband of 22 years might leave her because of it.

When I queried her about her prescription drug use, she explained that her gynecologist had prescribed estradiol vaginal cream, a potent estrogen in cream form, to manage vaginal dryness she had been experiencing. She was also taking citalopram daily to help manage her low mood, something she has been taking for over 10 years. That's when the warning lights went on.

I checked her hormone profile through kinesiology and uncovered the cause for both her key symptoms. Amanda's estrogen levels were quite high, partly from worrying about and over-nurturing her husband and partly from the vaginal estrogen cream she had been using three times weekly for several years. This topical cream which is absorbed into the blood stream was enough to drive the growth of her fibroid cysts. I also found that her progesterone levels were very low, partly due to the traditional menopause-induced hormonal shift and partly due to the unwanted side effects from her antidepressant medication, and ironically this was the genesis of her depression.

As is often the case, Amanda's gynecologist did not connect the estrogen supplementation with her fibrocystic dilemma. She also failed to recognize that citalopram, although helping with some of the symptoms of depression, was also causing her sexual issues; directly through the drug's side effect profile and indirectly by forcing progesterone levels even lower than they might have normally been.

A topical progesterone cream regimen of ½ teaspoonful at bedtime on the calendar days one through twenty-five was instituted to drive up progesterone and to help drive down high estrogen. I also advised Amanda to stop the estradiol vaginal cream since progesterone supplementation will often improve vaginal dryness. Finally, we began a slow three-week taper of her citalopram in order to avert uncomfortable withdrawal symptoms. Amanda seemed eager and open to using natural methods to manage her mood and libido issues, and was quite compliant.

We had several follow-up sessions together after our initial evaluation and during each visit Amanda reported little to no change in her sex drive, although there was a modest improvement in her cystic pain. She was beginning to give up all hope of solving her libido issues and was ready to concede that perhaps she wasn't destined to have a libido in this lifetime. I assured her that was not the case and encouraged her to be patient, as it can sometimes take weeks to several months or more to rebalance a hormone profile that has been stagnated for so many years, and this was one of those cases. Still, Amanda seemed desperate and almost in tears when she left the office that day.

Then about six weeks later there was a knock on my office door. It was Amanda. She had a quirky smile on her face as she leaned in to whisper into my ear. Holding back a giggle, she reported that her libido was back with a vengeance and that she couldn't be happier. Amanda had finally experienced the pleasure of a healthy libido and was as giddy as a school girl to feel like a woman once again. Certainly, I was pleased with the outcome, but probably not as pleased as her husband.

LOVING SPOONFUL

Or in this case, maybe as little as half a teaspoonful of topical progesterone cream can be enough to restore sagging progesterone levels from any cause. If your libido is merely a faint memory from a distant past, don't give up hope. Rebalancing progesterone levels will often restore a normal and balanced libido. But be patient, and do have your hormone levels checked through kinesiology with a trusted holistic practitioner. And while you're there, take the opportunity to discuss all the libido busters in and around your life that may be affecting your drive. Once they are attended to, you too can "bring back that lovin' feeling". Thank you, Bobby Hatfield and Bill Medley for those inspiring lyrics.

HORMONE TRUTH:

Women, if you can't recall the last time you had a libido, your progesterone levels are likely out of balance and need to be supplemented, no matter what your age.

HORMONE BALANCING REGIMEN FOR LOW LIBIDO

1. Progesterone cream

For women still cycling:

Topical progesterone cream ¼ to ½ teaspoonfuls rubbed into breast, stomach, thighs, or inner arm once daily at bedtime on your cycle days 12 through 26. The first day of your cycle is the first day of bleeding.

For women no longer cycling:

Topical progesterone cream ¼ to ½ teaspoonfuls rubbed into breast, stomach, thighs, or inner arm once daily at bedtime on calendar days 1 through 25 only.

- Rotate application site every two to three days
- It may take two to three months or longer to notice full improvement of symptoms, so be patient
- Hormone levels should be checked through applied kinesiology throughout the balancing period at approximately three to four week intervals

2. Maca 1 dose once to twice daily with food, or as directed on the package. Do not use for more than four weeks at a time, take a one week break, then repeat the cycle.

Hot Flashes

LOW ESTROGEN CAN LEAD TO HOT FLASHES

The topic of hot flashes in menopausal women is perhaps the most over-hyped and misunderstood phenomenon in the hormone lies debacle. Why so misunderstood? Because almost every female on the planet is quite aware of the term hot flashes, yet few understand what that really means with regard to their hormone balance. Even fewer seem to know how to fix it, and the rest don't even know if they *should* fix it. Perhaps hot flashes are supposed to occur, perhaps they should not be treated, and perhaps there is a good reason that nearly every woman will have the opportunity to experience that oven-baked, stringy wet hair, damp clothing feeling. I would suggest they are right on all counts.

WHY ME?

First let's address the why? What is a hot flash and what does it mean to women who are experiencing them? From the perspective of this medical intuitive, hot flashes are a chemical and metabolic signal that a woman's hormones and literally *everything else about her* are in a rebalancing phase. It's a potent and unmistakable signal that your body is changing, that your perspective about life and your place in it is changing. Think of hot flashes more as barometer rather than a thermometer. Like a fever, when these hot flashes or night sweats occur they are providing you an opportunity to reflect on the past and literally melt it away, so that all that remains is the true core of who you really are, and the understanding about what you are here to do in this lifetime. As nice and esoterically glamorous as all that may sound, hot flashes are not fun.

Despite the wonderful spiritual and emotional opportunities that hot flashes may signal in a woman's life, there's no arguing that they are uncomfortable and sometimes unbearable, to say the least. Many women will say that they feel "warm" in the face, or feel heat or a tingling sensation radiating from any part of the body, often from the solar plexus chakra or abdominal area. Considered by some women to be the scourge of menopause, these hot, sometimes drenching episodes can disrupt your focus, zap energy, destroy sex, and pretty much suck the joy out of all of life's little pleasures. They can even occur at night while sleeping. We call those "night sweats" and when they occur they are very often responsible for bouts of insomnia. At the end of the day, no matter what you call those uncomfortable sensations, they all result from the same thing: low estrogen levels.

SOONER OR LATER

When it comes to hot flashes, most would prefer none at all, thank you very much. But like it or not, hot flashes do occur in about 90 percent of women who reach that monumental cycle in their life called menopause, typically between the ages of 40 and 60. However, a fortunate 10 to 15 percent of all women are the lucky few who seem to be able to avert all tangible hormonal symptoms during their menopausal years, including hot flashes, and this is most often attributable to genetic good fortune.

But a disturbing hormonal trend seems to be emerging in this new day and new age, with women as young as their early 20's and 30's being afflicted by the flash. This early onset of estrogen disruption has much to do with the fact that more women are using hormonal disruptive medicines than ever before; birth control pills and devices that don't just contain a simple estrogen and progesterone component, but contain more exotic and varied estrogen and progesterone derivatives. These newer synthetic ingredients introduced into the body of the sensitive woman often result in disruption of the delicate and vulnerable hormone balance you were born with. Add to this unhealthy hormone concoction a genetic predisposition for hot flashes, underlying emotional trauma, or any other lifestyle miscues and you have a recipe for hot flashes, a recipe we just as soon not cook up.

It's no wonder then that hot flashes are one of the top symptoms that drive women to their gynecologists. They want these annoying episodes to stop. And who can blame them. The truth is hot flashes are a natural yet often disruptive event that has its roots not just in the collapse of estrogen levels in sensitive individuals, but also in other commonly overlooked events in the lives of the modern woman.

COMMONLY OVERLOOKED CAUSES OF HOT FLASHES

- Hormonal birth control
- Emotional trauma
- Lack of sexual expression
- Lifestyle stressors
- Hysterectomy
- Hot foods and beverages
- Caffeine
- Excess weight
- Genetics
- Environmental toxins, including heavy metal toxicity
- Candidiasis, Candida yeast infection, or other infectious processes
- **Low estrogen**

HOW LOW SHOULD WE GO?

Alright, so now we've agreed that hot flashes are a sign that estrogen levels are low. This may sound like a bad thing but what I remind my female clients suffering from hot flashes is that they should count their blessings. Hot flashes are a blessing? That's right, a blessing. That's because in general, if you're having hot flashes you *do not* have high estrogen, you have *low* estrogen, and hence you are not at an increased risk of developing the serious health consequences that often accompany high estrogen. We've talked about these consequences throughout the book; fibrocystic tissue growth in the breasts, ovaries and elsewhere, and negative cellular changes that can lead to hormonal cancers, and more.

Low estrogen = hot flashes
High estrogen = fibrocystic disease and other
negative cell changes, including cancer

Although the traditional medical community may come away flabbergasted by this notion, I have found it to be true in case after case in my holistic medicine practice. Women who experience regular hot flash activity rarely report or present with fibrocystic breasts and ovaries, endometriosis, or negative Pap smears. They almost never present with the symptoms of Polycystic Ovary Syndrome or PCOS. They will rarely be diagnosed with breast cancer, ovarian cancer, uterine cancer, or any other hormonal cancer, because their estrogen levels have never been elevated for long periods of time. Why is this so? How did these women escape the throws of these dangerous and prevalent health maladies?

There are several reasons that this is so. Genetic destiny is one of them. That simply means your maternal lineage has no remarkable history for these types of health conditions; your mother, her female siblings, or your female siblings have not developed these health conditions because, simply put, it wasn't in their cards. It simply wasn't destined to be.

Another reason some women escape the raves of estrogen dominance has to do with how they handle themselves in the play of life. There is a group of individuals on this planet who were born with a genetically stronger constitution; essentially they are genetically programmed with "thicker skin". These particular individuals tend to be more emotionally stout and allow life's tough punches to slide off them rather than allowing them to "move in" and take over. They tend not to internalize and consciously ruminate about negative events, and more often than not do not allow emotional situations or past traumas to control them; rather they tend to process and release these potentially emotionally and hormonally damaging events on a regular basis, like a pool filter that clears out the gunk from pool water. These fortunate individuals have a tendency to be less negative in their mind set, and there is plenty of evidence supporting the theory that positive thinking creates positive health. And this is the perfect example of it.

TREAT OR DON'T TREAT

Menopause has been around for thousands of years, likely as long as there have been females on this planet. There were no magic pills or cures for the condition back then. Yet trillions of women before you survived and thrived without any hormonal intervention whatsoever. My mother, who transitioned through her hormonal maturation era during the 1960's and 1970's, and perhaps your mother as well, took no pills, had no hormonal intervention whatsoever, and simply went on with her life. Like her, these women didn't allow hot flashes to consume them or suck the joy from their existence. They just worked through it, lived with it and moved on to the next phase of their life journey. You can too if you choose.

Oh yes, hot flashes will run their course, eventually. Some women experience hot flashes for only one to two years or less, others for up to 10 years or more, depending on several lifestyle issues such as their overall emotional inventory, genetic sensitivity, diet choices, and their ability to process and release the byproducts of this lifetime, and in many cases, *other* lifetimes.

So, should you seek treatment for hot flashes or ignore them and allow them to run their course? Before you decide, consider this. The current mainstream medicine practitioners know and use only one method to manage hot flashes: potent estrogen in the form of pills or patches. And, yes, these potent estrogenic products will indeed stop the hot flashes. Your physical symptoms will be gone, but a new set of hidden and insidious symptoms will begin to brew from potent estrogen stimulation of the sensitive reproductive organs. And then the health problems will begin. Maybe not right away, but you can be certain that negative cellular changes will begin occurring within five years if not sooner, depending on your metabolism and your genetic heritage. Not keen on this option? How about plan B? Go natural!

A LA NATURAL

Natural remedies are available to ease the symptoms of menopause and can be very effective *and* safe in the treatment of hot flashes and other hormonal symptoms. Whether it's topical progesterone cream, black cohosh, chasteberry a.k.a. vitex, maca, or a host of other natural herbs, alone or in combination, these natural products have been used for thousands of years to help alleviate the discomfort and reduce the frequency of hot flashes, without subjecting yourself to harsh estrogen. These products work by re-establishing the balance between your progesterone and estrogen levels, and they work quite well for many women. There may be a period of trial and error before you find the right combination that works for you, but once you do, hot flashes and the symptoms of menopause will no longer be consuming you and controlling your life.

Yet there is a third option: no medicinal interventions at all. This method has been successfully employed by many a past generation. Work through the hot flashes by staying busy with things that give you pleasure; temper your consumption of hot and spicy foods, don't over-exert yourself physically or emotionally, and do your best to work through any unresolved emotional issues that are hanging on and free yourself from all situations and relationships in your life that are not working. Finally, on a note that may be a bit squeamish for some, don't forget to express your sexuality. Pent-up sexual frustration can often lead to an increase in the frequency, intensity, and duration of hot flashes, and other hormonal symptoms you may be experiencing. So start expressing your sexuality regularly and in a healthy fashion suitable to you. Refer to the Sexual Expression and Your Hormones chapter for more insight into this pivotal hormonal topic.

Not sure which direction you want to go? Don't sweat it. Pun intended. Trust your intuition and you will know where to start. But whatever you do, avoid succumbing to the "my way or the highway" spiel when you visit your traditionally-minded gynecologist. You do have options and all the choices are yours. Always. A visit with a qualified holistic practitioner who is versed in natural hormone manipulation will be a good place to get additional input and fresh perspective. And who knows. You may find that natural hormone balancing is perfect for you. If you suffer from hot flashes and wish to whisk them away, get started today.

LIBBY had just visited with her acupuncturist who worked several doors down from my office. Led by an unseen force, and certainly not by accident, she meandered into my office to discuss her unrelenting hot flashes. Although she walked in without an appointment she seemed desperate, and as it turned out I happened to have a small window of time between patients that day. She sat down in the chair and we began to unravel her case.

In her late 40's, Libby had been enduring the misery of hot flashes literally every 20 to 30 minutes around the clock for the last eight months, and they were getting worse. She couldn't even escape the heat at night, as she was awakened almost hourly with drenched bed sheets and pajamas when the night sweats kicked up. It would be safe to say that hot flashes were consuming Libby's life. This was one of the most aggressive cases of hot flashes I'd seen in years.

I proceeded to check Libby's hormones and the results were certainly not surprising. Libby had extremely low estrogen levels and low progesterone levels. Although these findings were in line with her symptoms, I felt something else was at play; something else was exaggerating the low estrogen response and the extraordinarily severe presentation of hot flashes. Sure enough it was about to be revealed.

Libby explained that she was a yoga instructor. She was committed to her work as a teacher and healer and had a devoted following of students, many of which had been with her for a number of years. She went on to explain that over the years she had developed personal relationships with many of her students, they became like family to her. But like family, the feuds and the misunderstandings began to rule the roost. She often found herself the middleman and mediator of constant emotional confrontations and bickering among her students. Some students even became disgruntled with her teaching methods, especially when it came to spiritual beliefs and ideals and to group leadership issues. Unacceptable levels of back-biting, envy, and jealousy had set in, all the while Libby was struggling to keep peace and retain her leadership role in her income-producing practice. As is often the case, this group began to control the leader, rather than vice versa.

Over time, these emotionally charged relationships and the stress that she internalized from them had taken a toll on Libby's energies, and ultimately her hormone profile. In this case she had a genetic propensity toward *low* estrogen levels, and that genetic potential was expressing itself in full regalia. As it turns out, Libby's mother had struggled with hot flashes between the ages of 46 and 52, and so it made sense that Libby would have the same potential to experience significant hot flashes, if all other ingredients were in place, and they were.

Although Libby was most certainly bothered by these unrelenting oven-like symptoms, I took the opportunity to explain that having hot flashes was actually a good thing, a hormonal sign that she was likely not going to have to endure the plague of *high* estrogen levels, including fibrocystic breasts, negative cellular changes, and more. She agreed to start on a progesterone/estrogen balancing regimen that included topical progesterone cream, black cohosh, and vitex (chasteberry) supplementation. Libby also agreed to a series of emotional clearing sessions to help resolve and clear the emotional baggage she had taken on with the negative group dynamics over the years.

During that two-month period of time, Libby developed the courage and the confidence to speak up and take control of her unruly students. She diplomatically and strategically put everybody in their rightful place, ultimately developing a hierarchy that allowed her to take a true leadership role within her work "clan". There were a few casualties along the way, as several students left the group, but as always, it was exactly what needed to happen.

Libby's hot flashes calmed substantially over the next six months, becoming less intense and far less frequent. At our last visit together, Libby was delighted to report that she was experiencing only one or two hot flashes a week, and that her yoga classes were once again packed, this time with respectful and grateful individuals.

HORMONE TRUTH:

Hot flashes are a healthy expression of your estrogen status. If hot flashes begin to control your life they can be managed safely and effectively using natural methods.

HORMONE BALANCING REGIMEN FOR HOT FLASHES

1. Progesterone cream

For women still cycling:

Topical progesterone cream ¼ to ½ teaspoonfuls rubbed into breast, stomach, thighs, or inner arm once daily at bedtime on your cycle days 12 through 26. The first day of your cycle is the first day of bleeding.

For women no longer cycling:

Topical progesterone cream ¼ to ½ teaspoonfuls rubbed into breast, stomach, thighs, or inner arm once daily at bedtime on calendar days 1 through 25 only.

- Rotate application site every two to three days
- It may take two to three months or longer to notice full improvement of symptoms, so be patient

- Hormone levels should be checked through applied kinesiology throughout the balancing period at approximately three to four week intervals

2. Maca 1 dose once to twice daily with food, or as directed on the package. Do not use for more than four weeks at a time, take a one week break, then repeat the cycle.

3. Black cohosh, vitex, red clover, dong quai, and others; either separately or in combination as directed on the package

- Professional guidance is recommended if your first trial of any of these products does not bring relief
- Some of these products can interact with prescription medications, including blood thinners. If you're taking a blood thinner, seek professional guidance before starting

3.

The Hormone Testing Debate

Before we continue our journey of truth with regard to progesterone, estrogen, and testosterone, it is imperative that we clear the air about hormone testing. What format of testing produces the most meaningful results? Which is more accurate? Are the results even relevant or valid? Should we even be testing hormone levels at all? Those are all excellent questions, but here's the most important question we should be asking. Are we using the test results that are produced to do the right thing for the individual? Let's find out.

GOOD AS GOLD

For years now, the gold standard for testing of most health parameters within the human body has been blood testing. It's been used as a health diagnostic tool for over a hundred years. And although it's a useful diagnostic tool for some health imbalances, in my experience it can be a very misleading tool when it comes to determining hormone levels.

When it comes to testing for hormones in general and the reproductive hormones specifically, blood testing has met its match. It's not that we don't employ accurate equipment. It's not that our vena-puncture techniques are poor. It's not that we can't produce precise measurements of a specific level of a substance in the blood. Actually it's quite the contrary. Blood testing and most forms of traditional testing have gotten *too* specific and *too* technical, and not general enough. We are able to determine the exact minutia of a blood level, yet we fail to determine that blood level's relevance to what needs to be corrected, or cured. Metaphorically speaking, blood testing often paints an accurate picture of the tree but not of its position within the forest.

In my view as a medical intuitive, blood testing and other forms of testing that require a physical sample, such as saliva, hair, or any tissue sampling, simply provides a snapshot of what's going in the bloodstream at that moment. Yet in most cases it is *not* a clear indicator of what's going on in the overall health picture. It is important to take a broader look at the whole picture rather than relying on a single test result to dictate a plan of action to heal the entire organism. In my world, that means taking all life factors and all exam results into consideration before taking any corrective action.

RIGHT ON?

With blood sampling, it seems we are spending too much time and money and putting too much credence in a single, super-accurate test result. Accuracy is great, but is it relevant? Does it have any real bearing in the health symptoms at hand? Rather, we should be asking *why?* Why is this result out of balance? What are the underlying issues that are causing this test result to fall out of normal range? Better yet, what really is a "normal range"? And is that normal range the same for everybody on this planet; a one-size-fits-all? I would suggest that the answer to that question is *absolutely not.*

For example, let's say I want to measure progesterone levels in Jocelyn, a 33-year old client who is suffering from difficult and painful periods. Her progesterone blood levels may indicate that she is in "normal range". But what exactly does normal range mean? Does that mean that her progesterone levels are normal all the time? Or were her progesterone levels just normal at the exact moment we did the blood test? Traditional medical practitioners would argue "yes, this is a normal level". They might also argue that based on the established range (established by whom and compared against what?) that Jocelyn's progesterone levels are normal all of the time, since this particular result falls into the global standard range established for all human women.

I take issue with that notion. First, not all women have the same genetics, the same metabolism, the same biological needs, the same emotional makeup, and certainly not the same energetic makeup. That means that what's considered a normal progesterone level for Jocelyn might not be a normal level for her best friend Cindy who is the same age, height and weight, and is having the same hormonal symptoms.

COOKIE CUTTER CONFUSION

Am I suggesting that "normal" varies from person to person? Yes, that is precisely what I am suggesting. As an example, I have worked with a number of individuals, who after running through the gamut of traditional doctors, multiple testing, and hoards of prescription medicines simply could not achieve the established "normal range" for blood pressure or blood sugars. In one particular instance this individual simply could not lower her blood sugar levels below what her practitioner considered to be a "normal" level, no matter what measure was tried, no matter what prescription was tried, including the use of various high dose insulin trials. Each doctor she visited insisted that her blood sugar levels were dangerously high and abnormal and needed to be worked up further. And they were. But they could find no cause for the abnormal results. This individual suffered no physical harm whatsoever, enjoyed life to the fullest, and lived to a ripe old age, despite having what the medical community considered to be abnormal test results. This individual had a *different* range of normal, not only for blood sugars but likely for other health parameters as well.

Please be clear. I am not suggesting that you ignore any of your doctor's recommendations or abnormal test results of any kind. I am suggesting however that what is normal for one person may not be normal for another, and vice versa.

There exists a more accurate way to gauge normal results based on the unique "normal range" of the particular individual you may testing. It is a non-invasive technique often employed by holistic healers, and when performed correctly is not only precise but also provides results that are relevant to that particular individual and their situation. And it revolves around the strength of your muscles and the energy of your aura.

APPLIED KINESIOLOGY

Applied kinesiology, often referred to as muscle testing or what I call "energy testing", involves gauging an individual's muscle strength when compared against a person, place, or thing. You can delight in the specifics of this holistic method of testing either on the web or in one of many books on the subject. Do feel free to explore it in depth as it can play an important role in detecting your hormone imbalances.

I have found that applied kinesiology, or energy testing, is well suited to test many health indicators within the body, and find it especially useful for the testing of all hormone levels, including the three key reproductive hormones, progesterone, estrogen, and testosterone. Why is it so accurate and so relevant? As we discussed earlier, it measures results based on your specific range of normal, not some international one-size-fits-all scale. Kinesiology is able to achieve these kinds of results because they are derived from your aura, your energy field, your specific energetic bar code, a sequence of energy signatures unique to you. And because no two women (or men) have the exact same hormone profile, this type of testing can help detect nuances that could only be differentiated through a check of your energy signature, the one that identifies each of us uniquely; hence the term "energy testing". In essence, applied kinesiology measures your "normal" against a range that is normal for you and your genetic and energetic makeup. This type of result allows the astute holistic practitioner to develop just the right treatment protocol to rebalance your hormones, as well as the rest of your physical and emotional being.

MICHAEL is a 62-year old gentleman who came to see me because he was experiencing new-onset symptoms of anxiety and insomnia. His medical history revealed no clues for his complaint, except one. He was taking the thyroid stimulant medication, levothyroxine, originally prescribed for bouts of fatigue and unexplained weight gain that Michael had been experiencing. When I queried him about his current levothyroxine dosage, he explained that his primary care physician had just received the results of his yearly blood test for thyroid function, and according to his doctor, TSH or thyroid stimulating hormone level results seemed to indicate that Michael's thyroid was still sluggish. As a result, his doctor increased Michael's levothyroxine dosage, and within just two weeks this new higher dosage ushered in the new symptoms Michael came to see me about.

I commenced my usual energy assessment which is part of my initial visit with my clients, and with one look it was clear to me that Michael was in a hyperthyroid state, likely induced by the newly increased dose of levothyroxine. Yet at the same time I felt that there was nothing *at all wrong with Michael's thyroid.* Instead, I sensed a moderate to significant mineral deficiency was to blame for Michael's original symptoms of fatigue and weight gain; more specifically, Michael was iodine deficient.

Using my applied kinesiology technique, and not at all to my surprise, I found that Michael's thyroid wasn't actually sluggish at all, but was now working *too well* and *too hard*. Where his thyroid function would have measured at a zero out of four when balanced using my kinesiology technique, Michael's thyroid function measured a three out a possible four on the *high side*. Using kinesiology, which specifically measures energetic results against Michael's "normal range", we were able to determine that Michael was now *hyper*thyroid. I also checked his iodine levels using kinesiology, and again it was no surprise that he was iodine deficient, three out of a possible four on the *low side*. As it turns out, Michael's original sluggish thyroid and the fatigue and stamina issues that resulted 10 years earlier were a direct result of an insidious drop of iodine levels due to malabsorption issues.

I immediately started Michael on a potent digestive enzyme complex, a broad spectrum probiotic, or the "friendly bacteria", and 3000mg of glutamine daily, all designed to help improve digestion and absorption of nutrients. We also began a slow and careful replenishment of his mineral deficiency, which included a moderate daily dose of iodine. I also suggested that Michael slowly taper off and discontinue his levothyroxine medicine as I instructed. He was more than happy to comply, as taking prescription medicines was not Michael's favorite way to deal with health challenges. The truth is Michael was "granola", a natural-minded and self-proclaimed health nut. Taking a prescription medicine was the last thing he wanted to do, but he hadn't yet learned the true cause of his original symptoms of fatigue, and at the time, levothyroxine supplementation as recommended by his traditional prescriber seemed like the right thing to do. In this case, it actually wasn't.

When Michael returned for his follow-up appointment four weeks later, I rechecked his thyroid function and iodine levels using applied kinesiology. Now off of his thyroid stimulating prescription, Michael's thyroid level checked in at a perfect zero, in perfect balance according to my scale of kinesiology measurement. Likewise, iodine stores were nearly back to normal for Michael's physiology, almost to a perfect zero, at a one minus out of a possible four minus. His iodine levels were on their way back to perfect balance. Most important, Michael was no longer experiencing bouts of anxiety, and his normal sleep-like-the-dead routine was back to the way it had been all of his life.

Michael checked in with me six months later, at which time he took the opportunity to hand me the results of his repeat thyroid blood test, the results of which suggested that Michael was moderately *hypo*thyroid, or in a state of low thyroid function. Neither Michael nor I could concur with the findings of this blood test, as Michael explained he felt perfectly balanced for the first time in years, and was experiencing none of his original symptoms of fatigue and loss of stamina. In fact, he confessed that he was feeling so energetic and vital he was considering entering a marathon, an event he enjoyed participating in on a regular basis decades earlier. It would be safe to say that both he and I were pleased with the outcome of the natural medicine intervention, yet I wanted to confirm that all was well, so I proceeded to check his thyroid function and iodine levels once again to make certain they made sense, that they matched the clinical picture of the healthy and balanced individual I was now observing.

Kinesiology testing once again revealed results that did indeed match the clinical picture. Michael's thyroid function and iodine levels both measured at a zero out of a possible four, a perfect balance through my method of kinesiology testing. As is so often the case, Michael's level of "normal" measured through applied kinesiology did not coincide with levels of "normal" measured through traditional blood sampling. Yet by examining the entire clinical picture and comparing them against energetic measurements of organ function and nutrient balance, we were able to solve the 10-year thyroid misunderstanding, and resolve several longstanding health symptoms. And you can too.

BUYER BEWARE

As within other professions, not all practitioners in the field of holistic healthcare are equally skilled. As well, having the technical knowledge of how to do something and actually applying it successfully are often two completely different things. Yes, one must be skilled in technique, but one must also possess and appropriately use their intuition, or their inner knowing to bring relevance to the testing, otherwise results achieved through applied kinesiology may not bring the intended or desired results. Insight or what we know as intuition is an important factor in not only achieving accurate results but also in utilizing those results in the appropriate fashion to correct the underlying problem.

If you choose to have your hormones evaluated through applied kinesiology, make sure you are working with someone who understands what they are testing and *why*. This may take some research on your part or a referral from a friend. In either case, it's important to do a little homework before you put the task of balancing your hormones in the hands of just anyone.

There you have it. Blood tests, saliva testing, hair analysis, intuitive analysis, or energy testing. The bottom line is no matter which way you choose to go, the proof is in the results. If your practitioner uses the results of their analysis method correctly, no matter which method that is, you should be feeling better within three months or sooner. If not, either the testing method was inaccurate or the treatment protocol designed by your practitioner was not correct for your situation, or in some cases both instances may be true. If you fail to get the intended results, seek out another qualified opinion.

4.

Premenstrual Syndrome and Hormonal Birth Control

Hormone lies start young. As soon as a young woman hits the age of puberty, she is susceptible to the harsh manipulations of their sensitive and natural hormone balance from all the possible disruptors on the planet, and we have covered a lot of them in this book. It is not uncommon for young women then, women who have just begun their very first menstrual cycle, to have difficult, painful irregular periods right out of the gate. Why do hormonal miscues begin at such a young age? It has much to do with the estrogen burden that is in our environment and in our society at this time. As we've seen, these estrogenic disruptors, including pesticides and other chemicals and environmental toxins, prescription birth control devices, plus the full gamut of emotional and energetic factors we discussed earlier, are lurking, ready and willing to wreak havoc, even from the very beginning of our existence on this planet.

The truth is, hormonal disruption can start from a very early age, and can literally begin at birth. Because, let's face it, the stressors of life, environmental, physical, emotional, and energetic are all around us right out of the womb. And if the *mother* has been exposed to these types of hormone disruptors during pregnancy, as most have, then the repercussions of those stressors can easily be transferred to the child in vitro. So as early as at the time of birth, *and even before*, an individual can begin to experience a variety of physical and emotional changes as a result of hormonal imbalances.

HORMONE PROFILE OF THE PRE-MENOPAUSAL WOMAN

- **Low progesterone**
- **High estrogen**

- **Testosterone becomes volatile, fluctuating rapidly depending on circumstances and emotional state**

It is curious and interesting to note that the hormonal profile of the pre-menopausal woman is literally identical to that of the *menopausal* woman. Why is that? Sadly, nothing really changes in the hormonal equation for females except for the biological age of the individual suffering from the symptoms of high estrogen. All of the same hormonal disruptors that are present before or at birth are still present when you hit your menopausal years. Hence these disruptors are equally capable of negatively affecting very young women as easily as they can affect menopausal women, and vice versa.

PMS or premenstrual syndrome afflicts millions of women in their child-bearing years; they frequently endure the ravages of bloating, heavy, painful, and irregular periods, accompanied by breast tenderness, moodiness, and more. Or you could change the name and the acronyms from PMS to *PCOS* or Polycystic Ovary Syndrome, a pandemic condition afflicting young sensitive women all across the globe. In truth, PCOS is really nothing more than an extension or exacerbation of the typical PMS symptoms; a more aggressive form of PMS. This rampant estrogen-dominant hormonal disruption affects ultra-sensitive women from puberty and up, and is characterized by multiple cysts growing in the breasts, ovaries, or anywhere, weight gain, acne, hypoglycemia, and more.

Yet most all of these same symptoms can also be found in the majority of *menopausal women;* we just call it something different; endometriosis, fibrocystic breast disease, or some other descriptive hormone malady. I call it estrogen dominance. At the end of the day, all of these hormonal miscues, PMS, PCOS, and menopause are on the same spectrum of hormonal imbalances, and vary only in their severity and their ability to disrupt the joy and wellbeing of the sensitive woman. And this unhealthy hormonal shift can begin at any age, and if undetected and uncorrected early on, the hormonal chaos created by it will continue life-long.

SIGNS AND SYMPTOMS OF ESTROGEN DOMINANCE

- Difficult, painful, irregular periods
- Acne, facial or full body

- Weight gain
- Bloating
- Food cravings
- Abdominal cramping
- Pelvic pain
- Fibroid cysts
- Tender breasts
- Moodiness
- Blood clots
- Cystic growth anywhere
- Depression
- Low self-esteem
- Edginess with emotional outbursts
- Breakthrough bleeding
- Inappropriate hair growth
- Anxiety
- Insomnia
- Attention deficit symptoms
- Abnormal Pap smears or other negative cellular changes
- Endometriosis

You can call it PMS or PCOS or any other abbreviation you choose, or in the mid-life years you can call it menopause. No matter how it got there or what you call it, be assured that estrogen dominance starts at a very early age and can wreak havoc on a young, unsuspecting, and sensitive woman. And there are a number of life factors that can raise estrogen beyond the normal healthy limits and create that notorious estrogen-dominant state known as PMS.

COMMONLY OVERLOOKED CAUSES OF PREMENSTRUAL SYNDROME

- Ultra-sensitivity
- Lack of sexual expression
- Genetics
- Peer pressure
- Work stress
- Unhealthy relationships

- Prescription medications
- Candidiasis, Candida yeast infection
- Food additives
- Food allergies
- Environmental toxins
- Sexual traumas, including rape
- Overbearing parental units
- Religious dogma
- **Estrogen-containing birth control**

WAKE UP AND SMELL THE ROSES

Sadly when faced with a pre-menopausal woman complaining of any of the above symptoms, pediatricians, primary care physicians, or gynecologists will often start these young and sensitive women on estrogen-containing birth control. Thus, we have exacerbated the problem by *adding* estrogen, when estrogen is already too high. And although some symptoms such as period regularity and acne may improve slightly with these prescription products, the long term exposure to these potent estrogenic agents can have severe and long-term consequences. Hence, an unhealthy hormonal cycle is born, and is almost never broken, and quite often continues unattended through a woman's entire life. And failure to recognize and correct this estrogen dominance as the culprit of these symptoms sets the stage for negative health changes down the road. And a long road it is.

Estrogen dominance from the use of estrogen-containing birth control often continues unabated for the next 20 to 30 years. By the time some astute practitioner figures out that this estrogen dominance is actually the cause of these symptoms, significant physical and emotional damage has already been done. That's assuming that a practitioner actually does put two and two together. In my experience, this rarely occurs. If it does, it's not until the pubescent teen is now in her 30's, 40's, or 50's, facing long term and agonizing symptoms of endometriosis, excess bleeding, severe depression, libido issues, or the most common occurrence, a plethora of fibroid cysts on the breasts or ovaries, or cysts growing on literally *any* organ. These scenarios left unattended often ultimately result in a hysterectomy, partial or complete, or some other invasive procedure that scathes the tender female reproductive tract.

Sadly, procedures such as these are often unnecessarily performed in women as early as in their 20's and 30's. In worst case scenarios, which unfortunately are not that uncommon, these unchecked hormone distortions can lead to breast cancer or ovarian or uterine cancer, and this can occur even in the early stages of life in genetically susceptible individuals.

ALL IN MODERATION

Another key hormone disruptor affecting women entering puberty is the delicate and very personal issue of sexual expression. As with any age group, and really with either gender, inappropriate sexual expression or lack of appropriate sexual expression in the years following puberty can lead to significant hormone challenges in the individual, as well as tricky discipline challenges for the parental unit. And chronic mishandling of these unique challenges in post-pubescent beings can create life-long physical and emotional effects on the individual in question.

Inappropriate sexual behavior in these hormonally formative years, either from overly promiscuous activity to the other extreme, severe sexual deprivation, can result in negative hormonal changes that can literally haunt a woman through all of her sexually active years. There is a fine line between too much and not enough that must be carefully demarcated in order to avoid any long term repercussions. For those parents raising these sensitive individuals, it is important to strive for a reasonable and healthy balance when it comes to sexual expression, as long term miscues can send the sensitive woman, or man, reeling into a world of confusion, hurt, and in some cases sexual and emotional reclusion. Certainly, the parental unit will have the final say on how to manage this important area in the life of a young woman, yet I urge you to weigh all the potential outcomes carefully.

BEVERLY is a gentle and overweight 18-year old that was referred to my office by her mother, who was quite concerned about her young daughter's deteriorating health. Her mother also expressed concern about her daughter's extreme aversion to discussing anything related to her romantic relationships or sexual matters with her. That topic was completely off limits. And although modesty, innate introversion, or feelings of shame or guilt are often the reasons behind this not-so-uncommon behavior, I felt there was something else in the works. One look and I could see and sense a severe hormone disruption was brewing within.

Despite the fact that she was eating well and exercising regularly, Beverly was experiencing difficult and irregular periods with heavy clotting, severe facial acne and facial hair growth, bloating and pain, and suffering from dramatic mood swings and wild food cravings. Her gynecologist was quite concerned about the severity of these symptoms and the fact that they had continued unabated despite several years of traditional treatment methods to correct them; so much so there was even talk about surgical procedures to remove some of the damaged tissue. Understandably, Beverly was near tears when we began to discuss her situation. I took a few moments to reassure her that these symptoms could be reversed, and soon the tears dried.

It didn't take but a moment for me to see the clear picture. I was dealing with an ultra-sensitive, ultra-gifted, ultra-responsible young woman, who was most certainly having a difficult time fitting in this society. Hers was a clear cut and severe case of Polycystic Ovary Syndrome, or PCOS, a classic ultra-sensitive hormonal condition.

This was quickly and clearly confirmed once I checked Beverly's hormone status. Indeed, through applied kinesiology I discovered that she had a severe deficiency of progesterone, and a severe excess of estrogen and testosterone, all of which were responsible for the entire clinical picture she and now I were now facing. Although Beverly was not currently taking estrogen-containing birth control, she had been on a six-month course of these birth control pills several years prior. Because of Beverly's sensitivity to so many things on the planet that brief past exposure to potent estrogen was enough to exacerbate the hormone havoc that was now in play.

A regimen of calcium D glucarate, DIM or diindolylmethane, and topical progesterone cream for her progesterone/estrogen imbalance plus chromium picolinate for blood sugar balancing was immediately initiated. Over a period of several months Beverly slowly but surely began to notice positive results. Her mood began to stabilize, sugar cravings became a thing of the past, and her facial acne slowly but surely began to clear. One of the most profound and welcomed improvements was the regularity of her monthly cycle, something Beverly had never experienced. No more heavy or clotty periods, and her cycles came and went like clockwork with minimal discomfort. The uncomfortable cystic breasts and pelvic pain also began to subside, although this did take the better part of a year to fully clear.

But there was still more positive news yet to come from this hormonal revival, in fact there was a rainbow behind this particular storm clearing. Not only were Beverly's severe hormonal symptoms resolved, but with her hormones now properly balanced, she suddenly found herself more interested in the opposite sex and the proposition of dating. This revelation was soon followed by an open and healthy dialogue between her and her mother regarding all facets of the dating and mating process; a comfortable dialogue which made both parties feel quite content.

Beverly's dramatic symptomatic improvement led her to swear off the use of all estrogenic substances from that point on. With guidance from her mother and an astute open-minded gynecologist, Beverly settled on a non-hormonal birth control regimen that was perfect for her lifestyle and her unique sensitivity. More important, her new-found energy and inspiration motivated her to undertake a lengthy and thorough clearing of all of the hormone and energetic disruptors in her life, a smart and worthwhile endeavor for her to pursue. When we last visited, Beverly was excited to report that she had rekindled her intense passion for the arts, and today is well on her way to hanging her work in some of the most prestigious galleries in her home state.

BIRTH CONTROL IN THE SENSITIVE WOMAN

Let's face it. Young women need to have contraceptive options. That said, the use of estrogen-containing birth control pills and devices can have negative health ramifications long term, especially in ultra-sensitive females. Even a single or short term exposure to estrogen containing substances can set off a hormonal/metabolic cascade of events that can lead to PCOS and other estrogen dominant situations. It's no wonder then that making safe and sensible birth control choices in the sensitive woman can be a challenge.

Because of their potential for inducing negative and sometimes irreversible hormonal havoc, hormonal-based birth control options should be carefully weighed before starting any contraceptive measures. The traditional health care system and its practitioners routinely dispense estrogen-progesterone contraceptive products on the first request, often without consideration or regard for the long-term hormonal disruption that might ensure at any time thereafter. That's why it's important to open and develop a frank dialogue with your gynecologist about these concerns *before* the prescription is written.

PREG ME NOT

There are a number of contraceptive alternatives to the traditional hormonal birth control pill protocol. Certainly, the use of condoms accompanied by other barrier methods may be appropriate, although their overall reduced effectiveness in preventing pregnancy should always be a consideration. A prescription vaginal ring saturated with both estrogen and progesterone components is also available, but it should be noted that although used intra-vaginally, this product still secretes potent estrogen that will get into the blood stream, hence can still pose a hormonal health challenge in the sensitive woman. For this reason, it might be wise to avoid this form of contraception as a long term contraceptive solution.

So how does the sensitive pre-menopausal woman manage the crucial issue of pregnancy prevention? By making smart and informed choices based on all factors in her life, and by considering all the options available to you. One of those options is the progesterone-only birth control pill. Because these products contain no form of estrogen they will not set off the estrogen-dominant cascade of events plaguing the majority of women in this age group, or any age group for that matter. And although there are some concerns that these progesterone-only products may not be quite as effective in pregnancy prevention, in general they remain a healthy and often a sensible compromise for many women. The intra-uterine device or IUD is another reasonable option available for the sensitive woman and should be considered for women who are in stable and predictable relationships, and where other lifestyle factors permit.

Your gynecologist can review these choices with you, but I encourage you to do your homework and explore all your options even before you schedule your visit. In your discovery however, please keep in mind that from a side-effect and hormonal-disruptive standpoint, what may be acceptable and tolerable for one woman may not be tolerable and acceptable for you. Not everybody is sensitive like you are; hence your decision should be based on many factors, and not just cost or ease of use.

HORMONES FOR ACNE? *REALLY?*

While we are on the subject of birth control, it should be noted that many primary care physicians, dermatologists, and gynecologists have been trained to prescribe combination birth control pills, that is, pills containing both estrogen and progesterone, to treat acne in either pre-menopausal, and even peri-menopausal (those in the midst of it), or *post-menopausal* women. I find that practice akin to pouring salt water onto an open wound. Hormonal acne is almost always due to high circulating estrogen, high circulating testosterone, or a combination thereof. Why then would you want to add additional estrogen in this situation? Ironically, this appears to be a commonplace practice, one that can lead to unhealthy consequences long term. If you're serious about getting acne under control and keeping it there, balance your hormones first under the guidance of a qualified practitioner.

In the meanwhile, natural non-hormonal interventions are also available to help get those skin eruptions under control. Start by cleaning the skin thoroughly twice daily with a gentle hypo-allergenic facial cleanser. Take inositol 500 to 1000mg several times daily to help balance high testosterone levels. Adding zinc 50mg daily, buffered vitamin C up to 5000mg daily to tummy tolerance in divided doses will also help reduce acne outbreaks over time. And there are a number of other safe, natural remedies available to clear acne resulting from hormonal causes, or from any cause, if you look for them. By the way, dabbing milk of magnesia on the acne lesions once to twice daily is also effective. Yes, it does work for many women and is quite safe and inexpensive.

Whatever natural remedy you use, do all you can to avoid hormone-containing substances to manage acne breakouts. You and your face can do better than that.

HAVE A LITTLE CHAT

The key to preventing hormonal disturbances such as PMS and PCOS, and any other estrogen-dominant state starts with a frank and candid conversation with your gynecologist. This dialogue should focus on your concern about estrogen dominance and the health concerns this poses for woman of all ages. When it comes to birth control options, urge your practitioner to consider a progesterone-only form of the birth control pill if the oral pill is the choice you make. Many gynecologists will argue that progesterone-only pills are not quite as effective or that they may themselves create hormonal imbalances. I would argue that no hormone imbalance could be worse than an estrogen-dominant state and no choice could be worse than giving estrogen in any form to the sensitive woman, or any woman for that matter. At the end of the day which substances you intentionally put in your body is your choice. Make sure these choices are fully evaluated and informed choices, and are not based on hormone lies.

YOU TOO CAN PREVENT PMS NATURALLY

Life can be challenging. Achieving perfect hormone balance can be tricky, and almost always is. But rest assured that natural methods are available to make the reproductive years comfortable and pleasant. You don't have to suffer from ravages of PMS, PCOS, or any other unhealthy acronyms. Seek out and engage the services of holistic practitioners in your area who have the expertise and the know-how to manage the sensitive hormonal balance of the ultra-sensitive woman, and you too can achieve hormonal bliss!

HORMONE TRUTH:

Hormonal birth control products that contain estrogen increase the potential for creating many of the symptoms and health challenges of estrogen dominance, including PMS and PCOS, and should be avoided when possible.

HORMONE BALANCING REGIMEN FOR PMS

1. Progesterone cream

For women still cycling:

Topical progesterone cream ¼ to ½ teaspoonfuls rubbed into breast, stomach, thighs, or inner arm once to twice daily on your cycle days 12 through 26. The first day of your cycle is the first day of bleeding.

<u>For women not currently cycling:</u>

Topical progesterone cream ¼ to ½ teaspoonfuls rubbed into breast, stomach, thighs, or inner arm once daily at bedtime on calendar days 1 through 21 only, or until the cycle resumes. If you sense your period is about to start, stop using the cream and allow the period to fully complete. Once your cycle becomes regular again, resume the cycling regimen above.

- Rotate application site every two to three days
- It may take two to three months or longer to notice full improvement of symptoms, so be patient
- Hormone levels should be checked through applied kinesiology throughout the balancing period at approximately three to four week intervals

2. Inositol 500 to 1000mg two to four times daily to balance testosterone levels and help manage acne breakouts

- May cause excess drowsiness in higher doses in sensitive individuals
- Inositol is not addictive and may be used on a continuous basis indefinitely

3. Magnesium 150 to 600mg daily in divided doses with meals to help with bloating and cramping

5.

Polycystic Ovary Syndrome: PCOS

If you're a woman reading this material, please pay close attention to this chapter. Why, you ask? That's because PCOS or Polycystic Ovary Syndrome is one of the most prevalent, overlooked, and undiagnosed hormonal issues on earth. To make matters worse, if PCOS is actually diagnosed through a perceptive traditional healthcare practitioner, the treatment options he or she offers do *not* address the underlying causes. Left untreated, as it usually is, this pandemic hormonal disruption will create physical and emotional symptoms that can make your life experience far less enjoyable.

So what exactly is PCOS, and what are the underlying causes?

Over the past several decades, PCOS has developed into a world-wide pandemic among hormonally active women. In my experience this condition seems to be most prevalent among women who are emotionally sensitive, or those females who I refer to as *ultra-sensitive*. What do I mean by ultra-sensitive? For a detailed examination of this poorly understood notion, I encourage you to read my book "You Are Sensitive!" There you will learn that not all individuals on this planet are wired in the same way. Individuals who are ultra-sensitive, both male and female, are exceptionally sensitive to most every environmental exposure in the world, including environmental toxins and chemicals, foods, the energies of other people, EMF energy from electronics, and much more. And the reproductive hormones are no exception. As with all the other organs and glands within the physical being, the reproductive hormones and thyroid hormones in ultra-sensitives are much more easily disrupted. If you suffer from the symptoms of PCOS, you are one of them.

SIGNS AND SYMPTOMS OF POLYCYSTIC OVARY SYNDROME

- Fibrocystic breasts with or without pain and tenderness

- Ovarian cysts with or without pelvic or back pain and tenderness
- Weight gain
- Viral infections, including Epstein Barr
- Blood sugar swings, especially hypoglycemia
- Acne, facial or full body
- Eating disorders
- Candida or other yeast infections
- Unpredictable libido, low alternating with high
- Edginess
- Difficult, irregular, or absent menstrual cycles
- Moodiness
- Insomnia
- Hair growth on face, breasts, or other unwanted areas

METABOLIC CHAOS

What exactly is going on within the body to create such an uncomfortable and often disabling syndrome of symptoms? Simply put, PCOS is the over stimulation of the reproductive organs and tissues due to **excess circulating estrogen and testosterone**. But elevated estrogen and testosterone levels are only part of the picture. Low progesterone levels are also part of the overall clinical picture, which coincidentally is not very pretty.

Over time the imbalance of these three key hormones come together to dramatically affect the entire metabolic system of sensitive and susceptible females, including the disruption of cortisol levels, blood sugars, microbial balance, and more; not to mention a complete upheaval of the reproductive system. This level of hormonal disruption can have deep-seated physical and emotional repercussions that can last a lifetime if not corrected, leading to sexual dysfunction, unpredictable menses, inappropriate food cravings, unhealthy mood swings, and other life miscues any female would just as soon avoid.

HORMONE PROFILE OF POLYCYSTIC OVARY SYNDROME

- **Low progesterone**
- **High estrogen**
- **High testosterone**

Sadly, millions of women across the globe are running around with just such a hormone profile, and most have no idea what's really going on inside of them. Most of these individuals go about their lives, miserable and uncomfortable, suffering in silence from the myriad of symptoms that can occur as a result of this precarious and peculiar hormonal conundrum. They often present to their traditional gynecologist or internal medicine doctor with unexplained weight gain, severe acne on the face and torso, food cravings, mood swings, edginess, and difficult, absent or irregular periods. In too many cases the whole PCOS picture goes unnoticed. And rather than look at all the symptoms together as a syndrome and correct the hormonal miscues that created it, many traditional practitioners will simply prescribe medications to treat the symptoms individually; antidepressants, anti-diabetic medicine, anti-anxiety and sleeping medicines and others are often doled out simply to cover them up.

None of these prescription medicines address the direct cause of the condition, which is essentially hormone hell. Instead, by employing these allopathic symptomatic treatments, the opportunity to uncover and deal with the actual hormone imbalance at hand is lost. Ironically, most PCOS patients are prescribed hormonal birth control pills or patches to control the symptoms and this practice is not only inappropriate, it is dangerous; dangerous because the estrogen component in these products will not only *not* improve the hormone miscues, it will raise estrogen levels even higher, making symptoms even worse and creating a gateway for serious hormonally-induced cell changes down the road, including breast cancer and ovarian cancer. This scenario should be avoided at all costs.

PCOS ISN'T PICKY

After years of working with hormonally imbalanced women, I began to notice a disconcerting trend. Nearly every woman from the age of puberty and up seemed to have the same classic PCOS hormone profile; low progesterone, high estrogen, and high testosterone. It wasn't just the teens and twenty-somethings that were suffering from PCOS as mainstream thinking might suggest. Women of *all* ages were showing up with similar symptoms and similar complaints.

In fact, if you're a woman suffering from *any* of the symptoms listed above you likely have Polycystic Ovary Syndrome. But before you begin to panic, please understand that this tricky and all-too-common hormonal conundrum can be managed successfully using natural medicines and holistic techniques. In fact, in my experience, women who faithfully comply with the protocol employed in *my* practice will find that most if not all symptoms will start to clear within six months or less. As always, each case is different and there are no guarantees in life or any facet of it, but do know this. If you suffer from PCOS, natural help is available when you reach out for it. And you can be assured you are not alone in your plight. Even though other women in your life circle may not discuss their hormonal symptoms with you, women with PCOS are likely all around you and most have no idea what's brewing inside.

So which group of women is most susceptible to developing PCOS? Any sensitive woman of any age group, from any culture, from anywhere in the world is prone to this profound hormonal disruption, especially when other life factors are also in play.

COMMONLY OVERLOOKED CAUSES FOR POLYCYSTIC OVARY SYNDROME

- Ultra-sensitivity
- Over-nurturing others and under-nurturing of self
- Poor nutrition
- Overly passionate and over-compassionate women
- Emotional stifling
- Lifestyle stressors
- Iodine deficiency
- Food ingredients and food allergies
- Prescription hormonal medicines, including birth control
- Genetic history
- Lack of creative expression
- Lack of sexual expression
- Sexual trauma, present or past life
- Exposure to environmental toxins, including estrogen mimickers
- **Low progesterone**
- **High estrogen**
- **High testosterone**

Upon close examination, a keen holistic practitioner will note an intriguing common denominator among women who present with the symptoms of PCOS. These women are typically deeply compassionate, even if this trait has been stifled by life circumstance, and are typically emotionally fragile individuals. For that reason, treatment methods for PCOS should not only include a natural medicine regimen that addresses the hormone imbalances, but one that also helps achieve emotional stability. One will recall that all physical imbalances first begin in the emotional state. And the hormonal disruption known as PCOS is a shining example of this notion in motion. Hence emotional and energetic clearing should be considered a key component in the PCOS treatment arsenal.

ELYSE is a 22-year old woman who showed up in my office complaining of irregular periods and hair growth on her face. At first glance hers seemed to be a routine hormonal imbalance caused by what I refer to as "hormone blossoming" or hormone maturation, the shift from puberty to womanhood. But upon further examination of this young woman's energy field, it became clear to me that this was not a typical 22-year old woman. In front of me, was a very sensitive, highly emotional, highly evolved individual, or what I call an ultra-sensitive.

After a brief discussion about her upbringing and lifestyle, Elyse revealed that she loved to sing and that she'd been singing since she was six years old. She also confessed that she was overly-concerned, almost obsessed with her recent weight gain, a nudge of about 20 pounds that could not be explained. This was most disturbing to her because she was working so hard to eat healthy and judiciously, and was exercising at least two hours every day. Despite these healthy habits, Elyse continually battled with bouts of weight gain, unpredictable anxiety and mood swings, and intense carbohydrate cravings 24/7.

She went on to explain that her breasts were tender, especially around her period, and even worse when her period was due even if blood flow did not ensue, which was often the case. She had even noticed a hard nodule in one of her breasts that seemed to become larger and very tender around her period.

A check of her hormones using kinesiology revealed the hormonal culprits; low progesterone, high estrogen, and high testosterone; the classic hormone profile for Polycystic Ovary Syndrome (PCOS). Presenting with all the classic symptoms, tender breasts with verified cystic growth, hair on the face, acne, irregular periods, weight gain, uncomfortable food cravings accompanied by hypoglycemia, Elyse was the poster child for ultra-sensitive women with PCOS everywhere.

A modified PCOS hormone balancing regimen that included topical progesterone cream, inositol, a B vitamin to lower high testosterone, and several estrogen and blood sugar modulating products, was begun. It took several months of treatment and several adjustments to the regimen to get Elyse fully balanced, but in the end her skin cleared, her breast tenderness subsided, and her food craving began to diminish, along with her weight gain. Within six months Elyse had lost a modest six pounds, which seemed to please her immensely. Most importantly, at least from my perspective, she began to have regular periods where the necessary cleansing blood flow lasted for several days at a time, something she hadn't experienced since puberty.

I also took the opportunity to explain to Elyse how this hormone profile came to be. We discussed her ultra-sensitivity, her overly-giving nature, her intense emotionality and compassion, and how important it was to balance these within the other aspects of living, such as her job and relationship commitments. I also assured her she was not alone in her battle with PCOS. Elyse worked diligently on the emotional aspects of PCOS and followed the hormone-balancing regimen faithfully for several years. Once her symptoms began to subside, we tapered down her regimen to just a few essential natural medicines. Today she remains symptom-free, happy, and balanced in her career as a world-class vocalist.

HIGH ESTROGEN IS SERIOUS BUSINESS

The hallmark hormone imbalance that drives the growth of multiple cysts in this condition is high circulating estrogen. Estrogen is behind the formation of fibroid cysts that can pop up literally anywhere in the body. For this reason it is imperative that before making the decision to use estrogen-laden birth control methods, it is prudent to give careful consideration to the sensitivity of the individual and genetic predispositions. If family history reveals cystic growth either in female siblings or any relatives on the maternal side, hormonal birth control of any kind should be used with caution, if at all. Of course these decisions should be made in conjunction with your practitioner and any family member who has an understanding of the familial hormonal history. And paradoxically those women at the highest risk of developing PCOS are the very same women who will likely have to choose some form of contraception early on. Please choose carefully.

HIGH TESTOSTERONE AND PCOS

High testosterone is the second most important hormone imbalance in PCOS. Not that low progesterone doesn't play a role in the condition, it does. But a progesterone deficiency doesn't pose the same serious or irreversible health challenges as can high estrogen and high testosterone. High testosterone is the hormone behind the symptoms of edginess, and plays a starring role in the development of unwanted hair growth on the face and the acne skin changes that are so common with this condition. It is also an accomplice in many of the other metabolic shifts we see with PCOS, including high cholesterol levels and a permanent lowering of the vocal range. The use of inositol, a B vitamin family member, does an excellent job in modulating testosterone levels and is one of the key components of the PCOS regimen, which will be discussed below.

Complicating the metabolic chaos that often accompanies PCOS is the fact that unmanaged high testosterone levels can stimulate a hyperthyroid state in certain sensitive and susceptible individuals. In my years of working with this hormonal debacle, I have found that about 30 percent of individuals with long-standing high testosterone levels will develop a Graves' disease-like syndrome that presents with classic hyperthyroid symptoms such as rapid heart rate, increased sweating, severe weight fluctuations, anxiety, bulging eyes, and more. Is Graves' disease actually the result of unbridled high estrogen and testosterone over time? This is most certainly possible. At the very least you can be sure that high testosterone levels are a contributing factor.

HORMONE BALANCING REGIMEN FOR POLYCYSTIC OVARY SYNDROME

As discussed earlier, the treatment regimen for PCOS is two-fold. First, as with so many other maladies, it is imperative to process and clear any outstanding emotional blocks or traumas. With PCOS, this is even more

97

crucial since unresolved emotional trauma is a potent trigger of high estrogen. Treatment sessions including emotional counseling and clearing, past life regression therapy, EFT or emotional freedom techniques, and the like are pivotal in accomplishing full resolution of PCOS symptoms.

This emotional clearing work can be performed concurrently while the necessary natural medicine regimen begins to kick in. This combination of emotional and energetic clearing along with the manipulation of hormones through natural medicines often yields noticeable improvement and results within four to six weeks. However, due to the relative depth and complexity of this condition it may take up to six to eight months or longer to experience complete resolution of symptoms.

NATURAL MEDICINE TREATMENT REGIMEN FOR PCOS

Please note that the regimen outlined below is a basic regimen, and is often tailored up or down with additional natural medicines as needed to address specific symptoms or situations. Although self-treatment for other hormonal miscues can often be successful, due to the complexity of the condition, self-treatment for PCOS can be tricky and wrought with pitfalls, and is therefore discouraged. Professional guidance is highly encouraged to minimize interactions and side effects, and to maximize results. Your holistic practitioner should be consulted to develop the proper regimen for your metabolic state, and to monitor your progress along the way.

CORE PCOS REGIMEN

These products are not presented in any particular order of importance, and most often are used in varying combinations to achieve your specific hormone balance. Specific doses are omitted because they vary widely, depending on a variety of factors. Doses and durations and the proper combinations of each of these should be determined by your practitioner.

- **Indole-3-carbinole blends (a.k.a. DIM) — balances high estrogen**
- **Calcium-D-glucarate — balances high estrogen**
- **Inositol - balances high testosterone**
- **Zinc — heals cystic tissue, clears acne**
- **Flax lignan capsules — helps break down cystic tissue**

- **Nattokinase — helps break down cystic tissue**
- **Chromium picolinate — regulates blood sugar balance**
- **Progesterone cream — balances progesterone levels**
- **Iodine — supplements low iodine**

YOU CAN DO IT

The health condition known as PCOS plagues millions of women of all ages everywhere on the planet, and most cases are never officially diagnosed. When they are diagnosed, traditional medicine treatment typically addresses only a few of the symptoms and almost never truly addresses the underlying hormonal imbalances, and the emotional and energetic imbalances. But *you* can. Take the time to pay attention to the signs and symptoms of PCOS and take action now.

If you feel bloated, are gaining weight, have blood sugar swings and intense sweet cravings, if your periods are irregular or absent, if you have acne, tender breasts, or uncomfortable pelvic pains and you are between the ages of puberty and thirty-five, you likely have the syndrome known as PCOS. But please understand that PCOS is treatable with natural methods. If you believe you or someone you care about is suffering from PCOS, don't ignore the tell-tale symptoms. Seek out a qualified holistic practitioner who is versed in treating PCOS. You *can* overcome and "cure" Polycystic Ovary Syndrome and enjoy a long healthy and productive life as the ultra-sensitive female that you are.

HORMONE TRUTH:

Polycystic Ovary Syndrome is one of the most prevalent and under-diagnosed female hormonal miscues on the planet and unchecked can cause severe disruption to your metabolic and hormonal balance, and the joy of life.

6.

Menopausal Mysteries

The hormonal and life shift process known as menopause is probably one of the most infamous and notorious events in the history of womankind. That's because at some point most every woman on the planet will have to endure at least some of the uncomfortable and often annoying symptoms associated with this monumental point in their life cycle.

Although most women who reach this milestone event in their life have few good words to say about it, when looked at from a spiritual and life path perspective, menopause may truly be one of the most wondrous things that can happen to the female gender (*that from the mind of a male author*). It should be clear that men experience their own hormonal and life shift at around the same time in *their* life cycle, but we'll discuss that in a later chapter.

Menopause should be viewed as wondrous because this window of time provides women an opportunity to take inventory of their life thus far, to reassess their path and their life mission; and to set a new course for new adventures yet to come. And regardless of whether or not you view *your* menopausal years as glamorous or not so much, it all comes at a price. And that price is the often uncomfortable and sometimes unbearable physical and emotional symptoms associated with the hormonal shift that unfolds.

SIGNS AND SYMPTOMS OF MENOPAUSE

- Irregular cycle
- Vaginal dryness
- Changes in libido
- Fibrocystic breasts
- Fibrocystic ovaries
- Skin changes

- Vocal range changes
- Hair thinning or loss
- Unwanted hair growth
- Weight gain
- Irritability
- Mood changes
- Breast enlargement
- Sleep cycle disruptions
- Emotional volatility
- Fatigue
- **Hot flashes/night sweats**

HORMONE LIES

Most women will tell you that they dread the approach of these menopausal years, and for good reason. Few would wish to endure all those uncomfortable symptoms for such a long period of time. And how long *is* that period of time? It's as variable as the women who experience them. This profound hormonal shift can begin as early as age 35 in some women and as late as age 60 in others, and can last five to ten years or longer, depending on your genetic heritage, and other lifestyle factors.

Though most women have come to believe that menopause is that time in a woman's life when estrogen levels plummet and hot flashes rule the world, I have found just the opposite to be true. Although highly publicized and often joked about, it's not low estrogen and the resultant hot flashes and night sweats that plague most menopausal women most of the time, it's *high* estrogen, or *estrogen dominance* that is rampant. As we learned in an earlier chapter, low estrogen levels most often result in hot flashes and night sweats in susceptible women. This is true. But what I have found in my years of working with menopausal women is that low estrogen levels are the exception rather than the rule. In over 80 percent of the menopausal women that I have worked with, estrogen dominance, or a high estrogen to progesterone ratio is the rule.

The truth is, that when it comes to menopause, and truly at almost any stage of a woman's life, a far greater number of women check with *high estrogen* and the resultant fibrocystic tissue and endometrial cell changes than check with low estrogen and hot flashes. Oh, be sure that hot flashes and night sweats can and do occur in a good number of women during menopause, but I have found this to be a far rarer occurrence than all that media attention would have you believe.

Although hormones can and do fluctuate during the menopausal hormonal shift, the true and typical hormonal profile in menopausal women looks something like this:

HORMONE PROFILE OF THE MENOPAUSAL WOMAN

- **Progesterone becomes proportionately lower**
- **Estrogen becomes proportionately higher**
- **Testosterone becomes volatile, fluctuating rapidly, depending on circumstances and emotional state**

And this is an alarming finding and one of the most damning and damaging of the hormone lies, because all over the globe in the *majority* of women everywhere, estrogen dominance is not being addressed or corrected by traditional gynecologists or other practitioners. And the unfortunate results of this failure to act are the genesis behind the rising rates of breast cancer, ovarian cancer and other reproductive organ, and even *non-reproductive* organ cancers. Yes, that gentle nurturing female hormone we call estrogen when left unbridled can wreak havoc anywhere and everywhere on the human body. But this estrogen surge can be tamed, and when it is, the life phase we know as menopause can truly be appreciated for the pleasure and purpose it was meant to bring. And what is the purpose of all of these symptoms, and when can I begin to experience all that pleasure?

PAY ATTENTION TO THE SIGNALS

Menopause is a wonderful and necessary event in the life cycle of a woman and it comes equipped with a host of physical and emotional symptoms at no extra charge. But what's the purpose of all of these hormonally-induced signals? Why are they here, and what do they want from me?

Their purpose in a nut shell is to let you know that you are changing, and as such, other things in your life may also need to change. It's a signal that you must now take inventory on what stays and what goes, and it happens at exactly the perfect time in each woman's life when that change is needed most. Now that notion may seem a bit cold, a bit cut and dry, and perhaps even a bit idealistic for some. That's okay. You are free to decide for yourself what these hormonal signals mean to you, but don't think too long, or you'll miss your window of opportunity.

IT'S YOUR TIME

The menopausal window offers you a chance to look back on your life, take inventory of what you've accomplished thus far and decide what you still wish to accomplish in this life. It's also a time to rethink life priorities and responsibilities. For those women who have given their prime years to raising kids and husbands, or other lovers, or even if you've just taken care of yourself and your cat for a lifetime, menopause is the time to re-evaluate all those past responsibilities, and it gives you the chance to weigh the priority of each of these life events and their place in your life right now. It's an opportunity to embrace new emotional freedom and to begin to express your true feelings, your true passions, your creativity, and to live life to the fullest according to your full genetic potential.

That doesn't mean you need to dump your husband or lover, forget the kids, and take a job as a missionary in South Africa, although some will do these things and more. Menopause can however be a springboard for making new plans, taking new risks, changing careers, relationships, employment, and everything in between. It's a time for planning the *new you*. And you can thank the recalibration of your progesterone, estrogen, and testosterone levels for the opportunity. These three hormones are ultimately responsible for the signs and signals that deliver the message that something has to change, that something *is* changing whether you like it or not, and with or without your participation. Whether you choose to respond to their call is a matter of personal choice.

So the next time you have a hot flash or night sweat, feel the pain of a fibroid cyst, experience the bloating and headaches around your cycle, whether you still bleed or not, the next time you over-react when someone asks a simple question, the next time you complain about how tired you are, remember the true purpose of these hormonal signals. Someone up there cares about you and wants to get your attention.

NOW WHAT?

Sure, for some women the symptoms of menopause can be very unpleasant, yet I have found an interesting correlation between the severity of hormonal symptoms and the way a woman responds to them. It seems that these symptoms are the most bothersome for those women who fail to pay attention to them, and who simply ignore everything that is being communicated from within. These women who continue down their same old linear life path without even looking up seem to experience the most intense, the most disruptive and dangerous hormonal health challenges. Conversely, I have found that women who *do* respond and react to these signals and symptoms and take the opportunity to make some of the necessary changes in their current lifestyle, tend to have more favorable outcomes, are happier and more content, and seem to be far less bothered by the symptoms of menopause. They tend to be more symptom-free than those women who just sit back and watch life pull them out to sea.

Then there are those precious few women who seem to bypass all the overt physical symptoms of hot flashes and night sweats. In my years of working with hormonal imbalances, I have found that about 10 percent of women, especially those from Latin descent, tend to have mild to non-existent hormonal symptoms during their menopausal years. This genetically blessed group of women seems to sneak right through the menopausal years without a hint of trouble. It's almost as though they skip the whole process for some unspoken soul evolution purpose.

Yet no matter how you fare during your menopausal years, a decision will have to be made. Do we just sit back and watch menopause run its natural course, or do we intervene as society has taught us, and squelch the symptoms simply because they're disruptive, or bad, or wrong, or unhealthy? But is that truly the case? Are these menopausal symptoms a bad thing or a good thing? Are we being selfish and unreasonable if we choose to be hormone-symptom-free? At the end of the day, each woman must decide for herself.

IT'S ONLY NATURAL

As recently as your mother's menopausal days, and most certainly your grandmother's menopausal days, females did little to nothing to manage the hormonal shift. There was nothing *to* do. They had no estrogenic substances to employ until the late 1940's. Yet, herbal medicines have been around and in use for thousands of years and were used and are still being used by some cultures. For the most part, however, our female ancestors just worked their way through it, if they were even fortunate enough to survive until menopause.

My mother, bless her soul, took nothing and did nothing when the symptoms of menopause appeared in her life. On the other hand, she also failed to react to the physical and emotional signals that appeared in her life and as such, endured some very painful physical and emotional consequences as a result. She allowed her life of emotional pain and discontent to control her until the end.

So what will *you* do? Will you pay close attention to what your body and soul are trying to communicate to you during menopause or will you simply endure the discomfort and stay in the same mode you've been in for the first four or five decades of your life? Are you happy with the way life has treated you, or are you ready to make some changes in your existence? Only you can decide. Remember that there are no wrong choices, only different lessons. And one of the many beautiful things about life is that we get to choose our lessons.

Please don't rush into any decisions right now, but please *do* take some time to explore all of your options once you've completed this book. There are plenty of them out there.

SARAH is a spunky, lovely woman who showed up in my office one day complaining of hot flashes. Although only 41-years old, she had been experiencing uncomfortable heat flashes and sweating at night for the past six months. She had attempted every manner of over-the-counter products containing black cohosh, dong quai, and vitex and yet still found only minimal relief from her unrelenting and disruptive symptoms.

Sarah was a hard core holistic-minded woman who had survived her childhood only through the use of organic foods and natural medicines from an early age, and with the help of several gifted holistic healers. She made it crystal clear that the use of conjugated estrogens or other hormonal prescription medicine was absolutely out of the question. Of course I supported such a decision.

A thorough inventory of her hormones revealed low progesterone levels and normal to only *slightly* low estrogen levels. In some women this imbalance would not have been enough to illicit hot flashes and night sweats, but as I'd learned over the years of working with hormonally-challenged women, each one has a unique hormone profile and sensitivity, and Sarah was no exception. Even this minuscule deviation from her "normal" was indeed enough to create these hormonal disturbances.

After several trials of different combinations of the usual natural medicines in my protocol, Sarah did experience some relief from the hot flashes, but not enough. Complicating the picture even further was the fact that new hormonal symptoms including insomnia and increased irritability popped up, all of this despite the fact that we had completely balanced her three key hormones; progesterone, estrogen, and testosterone. I had seen a few cases like this in the past; resistant hormone and metabolic coding that was difficult to correct through any hormone interventions, but this case was different. Nothing worked, no matter which combinations of natural medicines we employed, and we worked with no less than a dozen of them.

Sarah's hormonal symptoms would not budge. Then one morning while awakening from sleep, it came to me clearly, as things often do in those twilight moments. Maybe not every woman's hormones are supposed to be balanced. Maybe some symptoms are not to be interfered with and are to remain unchecked in order to learn a deeper soul lesson or purpose. Maybe, just maybe, in this case I was meddling where I shouldn't be.

I'd always wondered about my role as a healer in this lifetime; stepping in, intervening with Mother Nature's plan in an effort to help people feel better. Was I really supposed to do that? I am supposed to heal everybody who shows up on my doorstep? This case reignited those questions within me and unearthed that deep-seated fear. I had heard and I had learned from many years of working in the holistic health field that some individuals are not *supposed* to be healed, at least not right away; they are supposed to go through their symptoms and illnesses as part of their life lessons. Was I stepping on hallowed ground with Sarah? Was I not supposed to interfere with her hormonal process? It sure seemed that way.

I spoke frankly to Sarah about my concern; that perhaps neither I nor anyone else was to interfere with the natural progression of her hormonal shift. Being the deeply connected soul that she was, she fully embraced that notion and agreed to leave her hormones be. Sarah decided to allow menopause to run its natural course.

Sarah stayed in touch with me over the years, and through those years she gave me the same report. Her menopausal symptoms continued to be mild yet quite unpredictable. She had learned to go with the ebb and flow of life. During our last interaction only months before going to press with this book, Sarah reported that all her hormonal symptoms had suddenly disappeared one day, without any medicinal intervention. Indeed, a check of her estrogen levels revealed that they were in perfect balance relative to her progesterone levels, an outcome that resulted solely from the work of Mother Nature. The timing of her hormonal realignment curiously coincided with her embarking on several significant and positive changes in her relationships and her career. But we both agreed that there are no coincidences in life.

Sarah had gained a healthy new respect for those beautiful and wondrous hormones, the same hormones that made her the strong and gifted woman she is today. To tell you the truth, I too gained a new respect for hormones, and for the gift of healing I had been blessed with.

TO TREAT OR NOT TO TREAT

This is a tough question, and for some a difficult choice. On the one hand there is nothing wrong with taking steps to mitigate the discomfort of menopausal symptoms. On the other hand, is it healthier to allow your body to follow the natural rhythm the way nature intended it? Do you go "green", or do you to take steps to interfere with Mother Nature?

Let me be very clear about this. There is no wrong choice, and either choice is generally safe—with this one caveat; if you choose to manage your hormonal symptoms I encourage you to make every effort to avoid the use of prescription estrogen supplementation to suppress these symptoms. This includes pills, patches, and even vaginal creams. It's true that these prescription medicines will stop the hot flashes by raising your estrogen levels, but raising estrogen levels can lead to unhealthy cell changes, and is not the answer to curbing hot flashes, or any other hormonal symptoms for that matter. Raising *progesterone* levels *is* the answer.

The goal of hormonal treatment during menopause should be to balance the progesterone to estrogen ratio, and this can be accomplished safely and most effectively with natural progesterone supplementation, either through the use of topical creams or oral capsules. At the time of this writing, topical progesterone creams are still available over-the-counter at many retail health outlets, and of course at the offices of many holistic practitioners. Regardless of how you get it done, work with your holistic-minded gynecologist or other holistic practitioner to supplement your low progesterone levels. This is the first and most important step you can take to squelch hot flashes and other nagging hormonal symptoms that can occur during the magical years of menopause.

In addition to natural progesterone products there is a myriad of other natural medicines that can bring you relief from the hormonal signals of menopause, and many of these medicines have been used for centuries. These ingredients can be found alone or in combination in one of literally thousands of different products available in health food stores and on the internet, and include such things as black cohosh, vitex or chasteberry, damiana, dong quai, maca, and others. Although generally safe and sometimes effective for some women, these herbal remedies can produce mixed and unpredictable results and may require careful trial and error to find the right combinations that will work for you. In order to avoid uncomfortable side effects during this process, and to assure greater odds of success, I encourage you to seek the assistance of a qualified health professional.

YOU KNOW

So do you treat the symptoms of menopause or do you tough your way through it? Only you can know which way to go. If you're not sure, spend some quality time with yourself alone in meditation and *feel* your way through it. For some of you this may be a new and exciting experience; alone time. But that is exactly what menopause is all about. Ponder and meditate on it and you will make the perfect decision. Until that time, make peace with menopause. It's what Mother Nature intended. It's also a gift and a sign that the true you is ready to emerge and make a splash on the canvas we call life.

HORMONE TRUTH:

Menopause could be the "change" you've been looking for. Managing the symptoms that can accompany it can be accomplished using natural methods.

HORMONE BALANCING REGIMEN FOR MENOPAUSE

1. Progesterone cream

For women still cycling:

Topical progesterone cream ¼ to ½ teaspoonfuls rubbed into breast, stomach, thighs, or inner arm once daily at bedtime on your cycle days 12 through 26. The first day of your cycle is the first day of bleeding.

For women no longer cycling:

Topical progesterone cream ¼ to ½ teaspoonfuls rubbed into breast, stomach, thighs, or inner arm once daily at bedtime on calendar days 1 through 25 only.

- Rotate application site every two to three days
- It may take two to three months or longer to notice full improvement of symptoms, so be patient
- Hormone levels should be checked through applied kinesiology throughout the balancing period at approximately three to four week intervals

2. Chasteberry (vitex) 1 capsule once to twice daily or as directed on the bottle

3. Black cohosh - use as directed on the package

4. Maca 1 dose once to twice daily with food, or as directed on the package. Do not use for more than four weeks at a time, take a one week break, then repeat the cycle.

5. Soy protein shake 1 serving once to twice daily in almond or soy milk. You may also substitute soy isoflavone capsules; 1 capsule once to twice daily or as directed on bottle. (Make certain you are not allergic to soy before starting)

6. Inositol 500 to 1000mg two to four times daily and at bedtime to help you sleep and to reduce anxiety

7.

Bio-identical Bandwagon

Of all the hormonal jargon that the female healthcare consumer might encounter at her gynecologist's office, this is the one that they are probably most familiar with. Bio-identical hormones. There's a reason for this. Gynecologists who are on their game and who understand the importance of hormone balance, *and* who are open to natural alternatives to potent estrogens, will often prescribe bio-identical hormones to their patients.

So what does that mean, "bio-identical"? Without getting into the techno-medical babble, it simply means that the hormones being used are biologically identical to the hormones in your body, which means compared to synthetic hormones created in a laboratory, they are more likely to create the same exact effects in your body as the hormones you were born with. That's a good thing.

GO FOR THE GOOD STUFF

When offered a choice by their gynecologist, most women will choose to go natural. It's not just about "going green"; it's about wanting what's healthiest for the body. That's what makes bio-identical hormone therapy so attractive to so many women and to many holistically-minded practitioners. So where can you find these bio-identical hormone products?

There are several ways to get these naturally-formulated products. Your local health food store will often carry several over-the-counter brands, typically in cream forms and often available in a convenient pump mechanism to assure the correct dose is dispensed. Your holistic practitioner may also stock various bio-identical hormone products in their office and recommend them as part of a natural hormone-balancing protocol. These products are most always prepackaged in standard dosages and formulas and do not need to be compounded or prepared, and at the time of this printing are available *without a prescription* in the United States.

The other way you can access bio-identical hormones is to schedule a visit with your natural-minded gynecologist who can write a prescription for you. These prescriptions for bio-identical hormones can contain variable doses and several types of hormonal ingredients and are usually custom compounded at a local pharmacy.

All of these processes seem quite simple and pretty straight forward. So what's the problem with using bio-identical hormones? Let's take a look at a few pitfalls you may encounter while riding the bio-identical bandwagon.

SELF-TREATMENT WITH BIO-IDENTICAL HORMONES

Don't get me wrong. There's nothing wrong with self-treatment with over-the-counter (OTC) hormonal products as long as you have a basic understanding of what you're trying to accomplish, and how to accomplish it. Your self-treatment journey should begin by doing some basic research on natural hormone balancing in books or in articles on the internet. Let me assist by giving you a brief summary of the information you should consider before you begin to supplement your hormones on your own.

First, start with a product that contains only progesterone components, and not other hormone modulating agents such as chasteberry, damiana, black cohosh, dong quai and others, at least at first. It's not that these other natural ingredients are bad, only that they can change your hormone profile in unpredictable ways, especially in sensitive women like you. This can result in having increased hormonal symptoms rather than the other way around. These additional products can be added later if needed, but I recommend professional guidance at some level before you use anything other than straight progesterone cream. Even then, don't be afraid to ask for help from a skilled supplement specialist at your health food store, or talk to your practitioner.

WILD YAM

When selecting your topical progesterone cream product off the shelf of a health food store, be mindful of the wild yam faux paux. Some of the older literature indicates that wild yam on its own can boost your progesterone levels. It does not. The conversion from wild yam into progesterone only occurs in the laboratory setting and not in your body where we need it. It doesn't mean your cream can't have wild yam in it. It certainly can and that's not a problem. Just make sure that you also see another ingredient listed with it: progesterone. It's absolutely fine to use a cream that has both ingredients, just not wild yam by itself. You will likely not see clinical benefits.

WHERE'S THE BEEF?

Using OTC topical progesterone creams is generally a safe thing to do, and if you've done your homework and have some of the typical symptoms of low progesterone, such as fatigue, weight gain, low libido, or hot flashes, you will likely see some benefit, that is *if* and only if the proper dose is used over the proper part of your hormonal cycle, *and* if you are using a high quality, high energy product. And that's a big "if". And this is where many of the hormonal miscues begin. And I have seen my fair share over the years.

What I have found is that nearly every woman that has come to see me to balance her hormones, and has been using literally *any* OTC topical progesterone cream, still checks for low progesterone levels in her system. Why is this? There are several reasons, the most common of which are the following: 1) the dose being used is too low, 2) the dosing schedule is incorrect, that is, she is using it during the wrong periods of the month, 3) the quality of the product is sub par, and 4) the length of time that the product has been used is not sufficient enough to fully raise progesterone levels. It normally takes two to three months or cycles of continuous use with the right dose on the right schedule for results to be seen, although in many cases we can see symptomatic improvement literally within days, and that's always nice.

But logic does not always dictate when it comes to choosing the perfect OTC hormone cream or pill. There is yet another factor that can influence how well any given hormonal product will work for you.

CHOOSE WISELY

The fact remains that even the best brands of prepackaged hormonal creams with the usual and proper potencies will fail to improve symptoms in some women. Why is that? Because despite how loudly traditional practitioners might cry foul with this notion, the energy or *vibration of the product* must match the energy or vibration of the individual using it. That goes for all supplements and even prescription medicines you may take, and also applies to many other aspects of our life. There will be some who balk at this notion, but I can tell after 30 years of working with individuals with every health issue imaginable (and some that are not), and nearly every supplement on the planet, this notion does indeed hold true. If your energy vibration does not jive with the energy vibration of the products, it will not work as well. It's that simple.

Suffice it to say that when it comes to choosing hormonal supplementation products, prescription or otherwise, some products will work for some individuals, and not for others, and vice versa.

DOSING FACTORS TO BE CONSIDERED WITH HORMONAL SUPPLEMENTATION

- Biological age
- Ultra-sensitivity
- Current hormonal level inventory
- Lifestyle factors
- Chronological age
- Other underlying health conditions
- Menstrual cycling, or not
- Weight
- Clinical symptoms

Using OTC hormone products is a mixed bag. If products are chosen carefully and used properly, the hormonally-imbalanced female can see excellent results. If the product chosen does not have the proper complement of ingredients, does not have the vibration match of the individual using it, or is not used properly, treatment failure is all too common. At which point you have two choices. You can seek out the services of a qualified holistic practitioner versed in natural hormone replacement therapy; someone who will help you make the right choices, or you can select an open-minded traditional gynecology practitioner. If you choose the latter, there are some things you need to consider.

TREATMENT UNDER THE GUIDANCE OF A TRADITIONAL GYNECOLOGIST

If you are a female reading this paragraph, there's a very good chance you could use some progesterone supplementation. Most females at almost any age would benefit from some progesterone. But before you run out and ask your doctor to write you a prescription for bio-identical hormones, you need to find out exactly which hormonal ingredients he or she is planning to compound into that paper prescription they are handing you. Why? Because certain hormonal ingredients which are commonly included in a compounded prescription can actually do you more harm than good.

Many traditional practitioners still believe in incorporating estrogen or estrogen-stimulating ingredients in these formulas, and natural-sourced or not, these types of ingredients can stir up hormonal havoc. While a healthy and properly calculated dose of progesterone can actually be beneficial, adding other bio-identical ingredients such as estrogen, or testosterone, or DHEA (dehydroepiandrosterone), or pregnenolone might actually make things worse. Over time, a compounded formula with estrogen, or estrogen stimulators such as DHEA and pregnenolone could exacerbate the symptoms you came in for to begin with. And you definitely don't need that. Just because it's natural and in a cream formulation and on a prescription, doesn't mean it's good for you. Before you accept a quick prescription for compounded bio-identical hormones, ask questions.

CINDY, a 52-year old woman was four years into her menopausal shift when she found herself in my office one spring day. She explained that she was having "hormonal symptoms" and seemed quite eager to get her hormones checked through applied kinesiology. She literally couldn't wait to get started.

Her urgency piqued my interest. When I asked her about it, she explained that for years she had been using an over-the-counter progesterone cream with moderate success. Her fatigue and hot flashes had subsided and even libido seemed to be livelier. Over the last year or so however, Cindy noticed that her libido was beginning to fade dramatically and that she was now experiencing painful and tender breasts during certain times of the month; this, despite the fact that neither her dose nor her dosing schedule had varied over that time period. What had changed was the brand of the cream she was using. Cindy changed to the new brand about five months earlier. Concerned that might be the issue, she had the foresight to bring in both products for me to examine.

The newer product was made by a well known and reputable manufacturer and contained all the right ingredients and in the right dosages. It also contained a bit of black cohosh, a common herbal hot flash fighter, but so did her earlier brand. By this time, we were both perplexed as to why she was experiencing different responses to essentially the same product; but I had seen this scenario plenty of times over the years. Some products just don't match the vibrational energy of the consumer and I suspected that was occurring in this instance.

Cindy's hormone profile revealed just what her symptoms would dictate. Her progesterone levels had fallen significantly and her estrogen levels were running high. Indeed, Cindy had noted that her breast fibroids seemed a bit more painful and perhaps even a bit larger lately. That's when I took the opportunity to discuss the concept of vibrational matching of products to consumers. And while I was a firm believer of this rather esoteric concept, many of my clients weren't so sure. I was bracing myself for Cindy's response.

She was clearly a bit skeptical at first. It simply didn't seem logical that one's energy vibration could influence which product would work more effectively. But she gave me the opportunity to prove it, and I jumped at the chance. I had Cindy stop her newer progesterone product and had her restart the original brand she had been using. I even asked her to reduce the dose by 25 percent. Being the pleasant woman that she is, she smiled graciously and agreed to give it a try.

Fast forward eight weeks. My phone rings, and it's Cindy, about as gleeful and giddy as one can sound over an electronic device. She was tickled to report that her vibrant hormonal profile had returned. Libido had returned, her energy was up, and her breast tenderness was all but gone. When she returned for her follow up visit that next week, I rechecked her hormones. No surprise to me, her estrogen and progesterone were nearly perfectly balanced. Last we spoke, Cindy continues to do well on the same progesterone dose, using the same dosing schedule, and the same progesterone product she had originally been using. Yes, "good vibrations" could be felt from blocks away.

ALL IS WELL

Bio-identical hormones are here to stay, at least for now. They continue to be a mainstay in the balancing of hormones through natural methods, and when used properly, with or without guidance can help bring the female gender to the peak of hormonal perfection. If you suffer from any reproductive hormone imbalance, I encourage you to consider supplementation with bio-identical hormone replacement therapy and you will feel better for it. Check out your options at the health food store or better yet, reach out to a holistic practitioner or open-minded gynecologist who is experienced in natural hormonal rebalancing methods. They can help you find hormonal harmony.

THE REBALANCING CRISIS

One final note on bio-identical hormones and the rebalancing process; and this is very important. When you begin to rebalance hormones that have been out of balance for a long time, generally one year or longer, or you begin to rebalance hormones that have been severely out of balance, it is not uncommon to experience a healing crisis. That means some of your original symptoms may get worse for a while, or that new ones may pop up for short periods of time, especially in those who are ultra-sensitive, or who have other organ or energy imbalances. Why does this occur? Because the reproductive hormones ultimately affect everything about us, either directly or indirectly; and when you begin to shift from one hormonal state to another, regardless of which direction you're moving, temporary physical and emotional discomfort can result. This is what I call the *transitional healing crisis*, and it can last from one day to several weeks in some individuals, and occur not at all in others.

These transitional symptoms can include anxiety, mood swings, food cravings, libido fluctuations, and more. Just know that when you're on the right track in the rebalancing program, you may feel what you may perceive to be "worse" for a short time before you begin to feel better. But take comfort in knowing that most women who begin a natural hormone rebalancing program will begin to feel better within three months or so, often sooner. That makes this important journey all the worthwhile.

HORMONE TRUTH:

Bio-identical hormones are the mainstay of natural hormone replacement therapy. But natural doesn't necessarily equate to "good". Some natural ingredients used in combination with progesterone can create new problems and solve none.

8.

Male Menopause; a.k.a. Andropause

In fairness to the male gender of which I am a member, I felt it important to address at least briefly the largely unspoken male hormonal shift sometimes referred to as andropause, or the male equivalent of menopause. Andropause is a very real and very significant hormonal event that typically occurs between the ages of 40 and 60; and like its female counterpart, heralds a shift in both the hormonal profile and the emotional inventory of the individual, and is often accompanied by a host of uncomfortable physical and emotional symptoms including weight gain, depression, fatigue, loss of libido and self-esteem, even hot flashes, and more.

But the fact is that andropause is rarely acknowledged by the male experiencing it, and even more concerning, rarely acknowledged by any of the health practitioners he may go to, assuming the male actually goes to one. Men are notorious for never asking for directions about *anything*, and will rarely go to the doctor for anything short of death. Andropause is no exception. Instead of complaining about these symptoms or seeking out help to manage them, men tend to just hold it all in and suffer in silence. And that failure to express these bottled-up feelings and emotions is one reason male menopause, or andropause, gets so little public attention, and why cholesterol, blood pressure and blood sugar imbalances, and heart disease are so prevalent in this age group of men. The male gender has been notorious for holding onto its heart-felt feelings and emotions at all costs.

Yes, when it comes to acknowledging the onset of male menopause, there is rarely any hoopla, fanfare, or media press, yet there should be. That's because the transitional years of andropause can ravage the self-esteem, productivity, and life force of any size man.

SIGNS AND SYMPTOMS OF ANDROPAUSE

- Loss of sex drive
- Fatigue
- Changes in appetite
- Weight gain, especially in the belly
- Hair loss
- Heart disease
- Anxiety
- Insomnia
- Depression
- Emotional volatility
- Crying
- Lack of self esteem
- Reduced productivity
- Introversion
- Increased need for drugs and alcohol
- Hot flashes
- **Increased suicidal tendencies**

So what profound and monumental event in the life a man could be responsible for such dramatic expression of physical and emotional changes? Just a simple tweak of the sensitive hormone balance.

HORMONE PROFILE OF THE ANDROPAUSAL MAN

- **Progesterone becomes proportionately higher**
- **Estrogen becomes proportionately higher and often dominant**
- **Testosterone becomes proportionately lower**

THE SOFTER SIDE

The heart of the emotional and physical changes experienced during the andropausal years centers around the higher estrogen/progesterone to testosterone ratio. This new alignment creates a dominance of the gentler, more nurturing hormones of estrogen and progesterone. What does that translate to for most men? They tend to lose their competitive edge and their aggressive nature and often become softer, more emotional, and far more sensitive than they were before. Because of declining testosterone levels, sex drive begins to calm and in some cases makes an abrupt departure, only to be seen again after weeks to months of sexual absence. And indeed, at a global level this is exactly what we are seeing. Men from all walks of life are finally awakening to their emotional nature and to their new-found sensitivity; they're moving into their softer side.

THE CRISIS IN MID-LIFE

For many men the thought of losing their competitive edge, their sense of productivity, and the thought of becoming "soft" can have serious and devastating consequences, leaving the once virile, confident, and strong man in a wake of uncertainty, apathy, despair, low self esteem, and often accompanied by feelings of failure and uselessness. And for good reason. After all, it's been woven into our genes over the millennia that the man is the bread winner and must be capable of supporting and protecting the family unit, and more. When that phase of our life has been completed, an emotional crisis can be the result. Many have referred to this pivotal period in a man's life as the "mid-life crisis", an apt description since it often leaves the man in emotional and often physical crisis. This crisis will lead some men into the stereotypical behaviors the mid-life male is infamous for, such as purchasing expensive sports cars and trolling for younger women, among other frivolous behaviors. Yet even more devastating repercussions can befall the male in andropause, like an increase in suicidal tendencies.

With few paying attention to the process of andropause and even fewer doing anything about it, it's no wonder we're seeing a rise in suicide rates in males over the age of 40. This unfortunate and undesirable outcome is particularly evident in those males who are ultra-sensitive, those empathic and gentle souls who despite their size, "macho-ness', or outward appearance, have a difficult time coping with these changes and many of the harsh elements on this planet. And the truth is, there are many more sensitive men out there than anyone ever realized.

I can tell you from first hand experience as a survivor of this period, (although there were times when I wasn't quite sure I fully survived), it leaves you questioning everything about your life. It shakes your core beliefs and forces you to re-evaluate your role in this world. In short, andropause makes a man feel uncertain about anything and everything he once was certain about; sexuality, life purpose, value to family, job, and more.

RALPH was attending a health fair at which I was doing a signing for my book "You Are Sensitive!". It was a wonderful event and I had the opportunity to visit with a number of gifted and sensitive individuals over that weekend. As is typical at these types of events, the majority of attendees were female, although I spotted a number of men of various ages and backgrounds milling around the room as well.

A middle-aged woman was next in line for the book signing. She handed me the book and asked that I make it out to her husband Ralph. I was most certainly pleased to do that and was equally pleased to hear that her husband might be open to exploring the material I had written about the sensitive people on the planet. I happily signed the book with Ralph's name in it and the woman drifted off into the crowd.

It couldn't have been more than an hour later when a large weathered man in his 50's stepped up to the table. Hovering and huffing over me, he angrily waved my "You Are Sensitive!" book in my face. This man appeared quite agitated; visibly perspiring, gritting his teeth with eyes big as saucers. To be honest, I wasn't sure if this guy was going to hit me, read me my rights, or both. All I remember is that for the first time at any of these events I was feeling very vulnerable and truly frightened. I quickly scanned the room to see if any security staff or other large folks were available in case I needed protection from this agitated soul. But before I could utter a word he growled in my face "Did you write this book?" I knew I was in trouble. But then I noticed the large tears flowing down the cheeks of this six-foot-five, 250-pound man. I breathed a sigh of relief, centered myself, and listened carefully and thoughtfully to the rest of his words.

He introduced himself as Ralph, and went on to tell me that his wife just handed him this book that she had purchased from me. He continued his emotional purge insisting that I had written this book just for him, that every point I made about being an ultra-sensitive person had fit him to a tee. By this time, *I* was holding back the tears. I was thrilled that I was able to connect with a man on this topic, as this was one of the key goals of the book.

Tears and emotions still flowing, Ralph explained that he never thought anyone could ever understand a man like himself. He thanked me over and over again for writing about this topic, for writing a book about someone like him. His teary, gracious, and heart-felt outpouring was overwhelming for me, and I never saw it coming.

I remember thinking to myself that magical afternoon, that if I never sold another copy of that book, I will have been content to have reached out and changed this one man's life. The fact is, I changed his and he changed mine. From that point on I was convinced that my dream of awakening the ultra-sensitives on the planet, women *and* men, was on the way to becoming a reality.

CRY A LITTLE CRY FOR ME

There are tens of millions of sensitive men out there who are now awakening to their pent-up feelings and emotions. They are tossing away the old stereotypes of the tight-lipped tough guy, the "I can take it like a man" image. Men everywhere are beginning to open to their softer, more emotional and sensitive side. We're beginning to cry more often and express our feelings more fully, and this is a wonderful and healthy change. In fact, I sense that it's becoming not just acceptable, but fashionable to be a vulnerable male, one who is not afraid of expressing his deepest and most tender emotions.

But surviving andropause is not just about learning how to finally express yourself. Like menopause, andropause is an opportunity to reflect on where we've been and what we've accomplished thus far in our life. Most important, it's a time to ponder what we'd like to accomplish in this next new and exciting phase of our life, and a time to discover who we really are underneath the macho man outfit. During this discovery period some men may actually admit that they need some help managing the symptoms of andropause. And that's a welcome breakthrough from the status quo. Men are actually beginning to ask for help; most often by asking their doctors for testosterone supplementation. Yet, although hormone balancing may be the solution to easing some andropausal symptoms, contrary to popular belief, simply correcting low testosterone levels is not always the answer, not to mention the fact that the use of testosterone supplements in any form can create new and undesirable health challenges.

TESTOSTERONE TROUBLE

The medical community at large has been quick to attribute all the woes of male menopause to the evils of low testosterone, when in fact this is not always the case. Like it or not, this notion has triggered an explosion of prescription testosterone products to flood the prescription marketplace, accompanied by a slew of slick television commercials to sing those praises. But is testosterone supplementation the safest and wisest way to manage andropausal symptoms? Maybe not, and certainly not in every case as the television commercials would like you to believe. It's just not all that glamorous, or that simple.

The use of these potent prescription testosterone products comes with inherent risks. One of the most dangerous of these risks comes from forcing the body to shift in ways it was not designed to shift, specifically by artificially and unnecessarily over-stimulating the sex organs, the thyroid and adrenal glands, the cardiovascular system, the nervous system, and more. More important, the random and empirical use of testosterone supplementation encourages practitioners to completely ignore the true underlying causes of these symptoms, not the least of which includes nutritional deficiencies, stifled emotional pain, and low iodine levels.

That's not to say that there are not legitimate uses for testosterone supplementation in certain cases. Such supplementation may be warranted for inherited genetic deficiencies or in men who suffer from severe and debilitating physical and emotional symptoms where severe testosterone deficiencies have been properly and correctly identified. In these cases, supplemental testosterone may be warranted at lower doses for short periods of time. As for the majority of the male population attempting to age gracefully and naturally, knee-jerk testosterone supplementation is often fraught with metabolic pitfalls, often creating unhealthy cell changes that can lead to cancer, scalp hair loss, high cholesterol, benign prostate hypertrophy or BPH, increased aggressiveness, anxiety, insomnia, edginess, and that's just for starters.

Unfortunately, many men receiving testosterone supplementation don't realize these negative, potentially life threatening changes are even occurring, since many of these changes will brew for months to years before presenting with overt symptoms. Yet some physical and emotional changes arise quickly and can be quite obvious and unmistakable. Sadly, in too many cases these symptoms are completely ignored or are incorrectly believed to have no connection with testosterone supplementation.

SIGNS AND SYMPTOMS OF TESTOSTERONE OVER-STIMULATION

- Increased aggressiveness
- Increased anxiety
- Insomnia
- Headaches
- Benign prostate hypertrophy
- Male pattern baldness
- Agitation
- Lowering of vocal range
- Acne
- High cholesterol
- Increased cancer risk
- Unwanted hair growth
- Prostate cancer or climbing PSA (prostate-specific antigen) levels

EASE ANDROPAUSAL SYMPTOMS NATURALLY

Despite all the hype revolving around low testosterone or "low T", testosterone imbalances are not the sole hormonal culprit behind those andropausal woes. As with the female gender, *estrogen dominance* can create hormonal havoc in the andropausal male. The truth is, if any of the three key reproductive hormones should be supplemented in men, it should be *progesterone*. Yes, progesterone supplementation *in men*. In many cases, supplementation with topical progesterone cream will improve the progesterone to estrogen ratio, thereby reducing estrogen dominance, and this can help alleviate or minimize many of the symptoms that men report during this time of life, including erectile dysfunction, enlarged prostate, and more. Although I won't address this matter in any detail in this material, topical progesterone supplementation should most definitely be considered in any male with significant prostate dysfunction, including prostate cancer, but only under the guidance of a qualified practitioner.

Aside from the natural hormonal manipulations that are available, there are several key *nutritional* deficiencies that often contribute to the disruptive symptoms of andropause, and these should be carefully addressed in every male journeying through this period of his life.

IODINE DEFICIENCY

There are few things more crucial to the vitality and energy of a male in andropause than iodine. If you are a male between the ages of 30 and 100 and are suffering from fatigue, low libido, low mood, sleep or endurance issues, low iodine stores are likely to blame. As with our female counterparts, this deficiency can be remedied through the use of slow and careful iodine supplementation as recommended by your practitioner.

Iodine supplementation should be commenced carefully and slowly and iodine levels checked regularly through applied kinesiology to assure that the iodine replenishment regimen is appropriate. Most males should start with 150 to 250mcg daily and work up slowly as directed over a period of several months. Unfortunately, there is a school of thought among some "holistically-trained" MD's and DO's, doctors of osteopathy, to start with extreme doses of iodine right out of the gate. I discourage this practice, as high initial doses can shock the hormonal and metabolic system and lead to hypertension, sweating, insomnia, heart palpitations, agitation, and worse.

Iodine supplementation can also be accomplished by consuming plenty of iodine-containing foods and through the use of iodized salt when salt is used during food preparation and dining. You can find a great list of iodine-containing foods on the internet or in the Iodine Enigma subchapter in this book.

B VITAMIN DEFICIENCY

This is yet another nutritional deficiency pandemic that affects both genders, yet I have found that the male gender can experience more profound symptomatic improvement than females once a B vitamin deficiency has been corrected. The B vitamins are a crucial nutrient needed to support and replenish the adrenal glands and the nervous system, and are involved in nearly every chemical and metabolic process in the body. For that reason, supplementation with the B vitamin can bring about noticeable symptomatic improvement within hours of a dose in some cases. Start by taking 50 to 100mg of a high quality B complex vitamin with breakfast daily.

These quality high potency products are available at health food stores or at the offices of many holistic practitioners. Most multiple vitamin products on the shelves of grocery and drug stores do not contain nearly enough of the precious B vitamin complex, and hence these products must be supplemented with an additional high potency B complex to be nutritionally useful. The other option is to seek out higher potency multivitamin products that contain at least 25 to 50mg of the B complex within them. Consult with a skilled vitamin specialist to help choose the right multivitamin product for you.

Always take your B vitamins in the morning with breakfast, and do avoid taking them late in the day as they will stimulate the body and the mind and may cause insomnia, especially if taken after 2pm. In many cases I also recommend additional and separate supplementation with vitamin B12, preferably in the form of methylcobalamin oral lozenges. Start with 1000 to 2000mcg dissolved in the mouth or under the tongue in the morning to improve core energy and stamina.

PROTEIN DEFICIENCY

Most people on this planet are protein deficient, and protein deficiency symptoms mimic many of the symptoms reported not just during andropause but also during menopause, including fatigue, low sex drive, insomnia, headaches, and others.

I can not over-state the importance of adequate protein consumption during the hormonal shifts of both genders. The emotional and metabolic stress that occurs during these key life phases causes us to burn through all nutrients much more quickly, especially protein. This can be remedied by consuming plenty of turkey, beef, chicken, fish, beans, eggs, nuts and seeds, with at least one or more of these in each of the three regular daily meals. In addition to the three traditional protein meals, I also encourage all adults to consider protein "grazing", which means consuming some form of protein every two to three hours throughout the waking hours.

To be sure, never skip breakfast or any other regular meal time and make certain that the crucial breakfast meal contains *plenty* of protein. Eating turkey, a beef burger, or salmon steak for breakfast is a wonderful way to start the day and a great way to vitalize and optimize your metabolism. Lighter meals that include healthy carbs like pasta, grains, and vegetables should be the core of the evening meal. These simple dietary changes will help improve your stamina and energy, blood sugar balance, clarity of mind, and your overall wellbeing during andropause, menopause, or any time of life.

Supplementing with a whey or other protein shake is also beneficial and should be consumed in addition to the regular meal foods, especially at breakfast, and then again at around 2pm each day. Within several days to weeks of improved protein intake, the hormonally-challenged male and female will often begin to notice improvement in many of those uncomfortable life transition symptoms.

If you are vegetarian or vegan, it is even more important to increase protein intake, both in frequency and in quantity. Additional B vitamins in the form of a B complex, iodine, B12, and iron supplementation should also be considered vital. Additionally, vegetarian protein shakes are also available for supplementation and this practice is highly encouraged. These simple steps will often give you that needed oomph, that core vitality you've been searching for.

ERIC is a tall gentleman in his late 50's who presented in my office with several of the typical andropausal symptoms, low libido, weight gain, and mood swings. He explained that he recently visited with his primary care physician who had ordered a testosterone blood test, the results of which indicated that Eric was low in testosterone. This finding resulted in a prescription for a topical testosterone prescription product, which Eric had been using for several months prior to coming to see me. All was well for the first three months, until Eric began to have difficulty falling asleep, and according to his wife, was more edgy than usual. If that weren't enough, Eric also reported having more trouble urinating, something he had never experienced before. These new symptoms prompted him to seek out my assistance.

A complete check of his organ and hormone status using applied kinesiology revealed what I had suspected. The culprit for these unwanted symptoms was high testosterone, which resulted from the use of the prescription testosterone gel he'd been using over the past few months. In addition, Eric checked with very low iodine levels. It was the combination of an iodine deficiency and revving testosterone levels that were behind the new symptoms that were plaguing him.

I took the opportunity to discuss the entire andropause scenario with Eric, and reminded him about how sensitive he really was despite his six-foot two frame. This emotional sensitivity was something I noted about Eric from the moment he stepped into my office, and didn't take long for him to prove me right. As I began to explain the importance of releasing emotional stifling, Eric began to fight back tears, and then proceeded to commence a well-needed full blown emotional purge. It turns out Eric, like many men of his stature, harbored unexpressed feelings of grief, anger, resentment, insecurities, and the whole gamut of emotions. As is also common, these feelings and emotions had been bottled up for decades, and I just happened to pop the cap on the bottle.

Eric confided that he was always misread and misunderstood by others because of his size. He had falsely felt the need to live up to the macho image that so many people had of him, in his work relationships as well his personal relationships. As such, he continued to push himself to be productive and to fulfill his expected role as a provider and protector, even though the need for him to perform these duties had truly left years earlier, during a different part of his life cycle.

I did my best to comfort and console the man, offering him the words of truth that I had come to learn and understand: Andropause is a very real life event that will eventually occur in the lives of every man, and that the open expression of true feelings was nothing to be ashamed about. I also explained that in this case supplementing with testosterone was actually making matters worse.

I instructed Eric to taper off his prescription hormone gel over a 30-day period. We beefed up his diet, literally, encouraging frequent protein portions throughout the day. Upon my advice, Eric also began taking iodine 225mcg daily before breakfast along with a 100mg B complex with breakfast everyday to boost adrenal function and stamina. After several weeks of noticeable improvement we added acetyl-l-carnitine 500mg twice daily to gently and naturally stabilize his testosterone levels. Within several weeks Eric began to feel like a new man, literally. His original symptoms subsided and libido was on the rise, something that testosterone supplementation failed to achieve.

After our discussion about his ultra-sensitivity, Eric devoured my book "You Are Sensitive!". He began to take on a new and healthy understanding about who he really was and what he was really here to do on this planet. This revelation helped him release that driving pressure to perform and produce, allowing Eric to focus his energies on oil painting, something he'd always wanted to do but never made time for. Turns out, Eric had always been a highly creative artist; he just needed to make space for it in his life. With his hormones, nutrition, and emotions finally balanced, the entire world soon became his palette.

I SURVIVED

As a self-proclaimed ultra-sensitive male, I endured a very uncomfortable transition through my 40s, and now into my 50s. I experienced frequent mood swings, bouts of needing and wanting to cry, and other unexplained emotional turmoil. Like the others in my gender, I didn't feel comfortable talking to anyone about what I was feeling – *except to my wife*, who was as understanding and nurturing as any man could ask for. With her support and compassion, I was not only able to survive these challenging years, I actually became more productive, more positive, and more content than in any other chapter in my life. She was there to listen, to encourage me, to support me, and to help me see my life more clearly.

I encourage every male who may be reading this material, or any female who is living with or cares about a male in andropause, to understand that this is a real event, and that left unattended can have devastating consequences for all involved. Men, if you want to survive and thrive during your andropausal years, start by acknowledging that it actually exists, and accept it as a normal and expected part of the male life cycle. And by all means, reach out to those close to you.

In my experience, these years can be the most productive and wonderful years of your life, if you seek guidance and solace from those who care about you most. I did. And I would have to say that doing so probably saved my life, in more ways than one.

SPREAD THE WORD

Now that you are armed with this new information about the realities of male menopause, I encourage you to do your part to spread the word to all those men who need to hear it. Share this book with your life partners. Encourage them to read this chapter, or if they are so moved, advise them to check out my book "You Are Sensitive!", a book that has helped many men awaken to their true feelings, emotions, and their softer side. What's more, if you know someone experiencing the symptoms of andropause, do your best to reassure them that natural methods are available to minimize the physical and emotional changes that are part of this pivotal life event. More importantly, love them for who they are; both who they have been and who they will become on the other end of this hormonal reboot. And men, don't forget to reciprocate. Women going through their hormonal shift need your love and support in the very same way. Why? Because at the end of the day, we are all craving the same thing… Love.

Be a shining example of love in all of your relationships and you will find that all the hormonal hoopla is nothing more than hormone lies.

NATURAL OPTIONS FOR MANAGING ANDROPAUSE

There are several over-the-counter natural remedies available to help augment and support hormone rebalance during this transitional period. But as with our female counterparts experiencing the symptoms of menopause, the question remains, should we? Should we intervene with the natural cycles of life by artificially supporting the adrenals, thyroid and the sexual organs with herbs and prescription medicines, or should we just let everything take its natural course? Ultimately that decision lies with the beholder of the symptoms. That's because so many factors in our life can influence this decision; things like relationship status, career pressures, your overall health picture, and much more. Only you know best.

If you do choose to take action, remember that it is crucial to first address and correct the key nutritional miscues we discussed earlier. If after successful iodine and nutritional replenishment that is verified through applied kinesiology, symptoms still remain bothersome, a trial of several generally safe natural medicines may be warranted and tried *one at a time* at approximately two month intervals each.

HORMONE BALANCING REGIMEN FOR ANDROPAUSE

MACA is generally safe when used by itself to boost libido, vitality, and stamina. Follow the directions on the label, but use this Brazilian herb for no more than four weeks at one time, followed by at least a one week break.

DHEA or dehydroepiandrosterone, can be helpful in restoring libido, energy, and mood in some andropausal males, but should be used only in low doses, not to exceed 50mg daily in divided doses, and only when testosterone levels are monitored through applied kinesiology. Because DHEA directly stimulates testosterone and other hormone production, it should be used cautiously, if at all, in men who have a history of prostate cancer or any other cancer in their family tree. DHEA can exacerbate or initiate the symptoms of benign prostate hypertrophy or BPH, a condition where the prostate becomes enlarged and/or inflamed, creating symptoms of painful and difficult urination and more. Avoid DHEA in individuals who are already experiencing such symptoms.

ARGININE AND ORNITHINE are amino acids that support and stimulate the production of our natural growth hormone levels. For this reason, they can be useful in restoring stamina and vitality. Arginine in doses exceeding 1000mg daily can lower blood pressure, so caution should be exercised if one is also taking blood pressure lowering prescription medicines. Arginine also stimulates viral shedding and may lead to viral outbreaks in susceptible individuals. Be aware.

ACETYL-L-CARNITINE is another supplement that supports testosterone balance during andropause. An amino acid that can improve energy, memory and mood, it can also help gently and naturally restore testosterone balance, improve heart health, and restore clear thinking, and more. Typical doses are 250 to 500mg twice daily, sometimes higher. If you are sensitive (and you are!), start with 250mg once daily and work up slowly. Cost can be a factor with this natural medicine, but is often well worth the price when considering all other options. It is one of the safest supplements of the group, with a great benefit-to-risk ratio.

PROGESTERONE CREAM can be very useful in balancing the progesterone to estrogen ratio in men, especially during andropause. Doses of 5 to10 mg daily should be applied topically to the testes or as directed on the package label. Topical progesterone cream can help restore virility, improve mood, and reduce the inflammation often seen with BPH, benign prostate hypertrophy, among its other health benefits. Progesterone, estrogen, and testosterone levels should be checked through applied kinesiology to determine the proper dose and duration of treatment. Over-the-counter progesterone cream formulations designed specifically for men are available through most of the usual outlets, and are generally inexpensive.

As with all medicines, natural or prescription, use these products for limited periods of time, a month to three at a time, and do take the opportunity to lower the doses, the dosage frequency, or take a rest from them completely once symptoms have been alleviated. Work with your practitioner to help you decide how and when to accomplish this.

HORMONE TRUTH:

Andropause is a real hormonal event that each man will experience at some point in his life. The symptoms associated with andropause can be managed through a combination of nutritional replenishment, natural medicines, and adequate emotional expression.

9.

Thyroid Misunderstandings

Hashimoto's and Graves' Disease
The Iodine Enigma
Goiters
Thyroid Stimulants: Levothyroxine, Desiccated
Thyroid Extract, and Friends

The thyroid gland is perhaps one of the most important glands within the physical body, responsible for maintaining the ever coveted weight management, our energy levels, mood and overall disposition, heart rate, temperature control, and many other crucial aspects of our physical being. Not that all the other glands don't play an important role in our viability, and overall health. They do. But few other glands control so many different facets of our overall wellbeing as this walnut-sized gland that resides in our throat, or the area I will refer to as the throat chakra.

SIGNS AND SYMPTOMS OF THYROID MALFUNCTION

- Fatigue
- Unexplained weight gain or loss
- Libido swings
- Mood changes
- Insomnia
- Hair loss
- Depression
- Enlarged thyroid or goiter
- Constipation or diarrhea
- Muscle weakness or jitteriness

- Increased sensitivity to heat or cold
- Anxiety and panic attacks
- Menstrual irregularities
- Changes in appetite
- Blood sugar problems
- Heart problems
- **Difficulty expressing one self, verbally and non-verbally**

THYROID SPEAK

Not only does the thyroid gland regulate so many aspects of our physical body, such as weight and energy levels, it also affects many of the unseen or energetic aspects as well. One of the most important of those unseen energetic aspects is known as the **chakra system**, an invisible and complex energy communication system that resides within each of our bodies. Although almost never acknowledged by the traditional medical community, the chakra system plays a vital role in our overall physical, emotional, spiritual, and mental wellbeing. Our body houses seven such major chakra or energy distribution centers with each controlling the energy and functionality of the organs that lie in that plane or section of the body. In this case, the thyroid lies in the fifth chakra, or energy center of our body, an area that corresponds to the throat. Hence the fifth chakra is often referred to as the throat chakra.

One of the key roles of the throat chakra, besides its potent influence upon thyroid function, is to establish and maintain effective communication channels, both in the sending of communication and receiving of communication. And this coincides appropriately with the fact that the thyroid essentially lays over our voice box, our vocal chords, the place where physical vibrations that result in our ability to speak aloud, originates. What does all this have to do with your thyroid? A lot.

SPEAK UP

Since the thyroid gland lies in the same region where the voice box lies, thyroid malfunctions can create difficulties in expression of all types, including communication of our thoughts, feelings, and emotions. Conversely, and more importantly, when we fail to communicate openly and honestly over long periods of time, when we squelch our expression for any reason, the energetic and ultimately physical functioning of the thyroid gland can be adversely affected. That is why upon closer investigation, individuals who have goiters or other thyroid imbalances often have "unspoken" or unacknowledged issues in their communication with others. In many cases these individuals have either failed to speak their mind over the years, or their freedom of speech has been squelched from emotional or physical trauma, or other fear-based emotions or events.

For some of you this notion may be a bit hard to swallow (pun intended), but I can assure you that I have observed this phenomenon over and over again in my years of healing work. It does hold true in nearly every case I've examined. If you're not expressing yourself in the manner in which you were genetically coded to express yourself, you will likely experience some level of thyroid dysfunction at some point in your life. The point is simply this. When your thyroid is out of kilter, your ability to communicate effectively with others, either verbally or non-verbally, can be compromised. And that's a big deal.

Given the number of critical aspects of ourselves that are under the control of the thyroid gland, including our ability to communicate effectively, it behooves us to take a closer and more practical look at how thyroid malfunction, and the misunderstandings that surround it, are unknowingly affecting you, and millions of others around you.

WHIP IT GOOD

In my experience, more confusion, misunderstanding, and metabolic miscues have occurred with treatment of thyroid dysfunction than perhaps with any other gland in the body. Why is that? Because rather than attempting to correct the *underlying causes* of low and high thyroid function, mainstream medical treatments have focused only on metabolically poking, prodding or stimulating the thyroid gland to work harder than it needs to, often creating new metabolic problems. Sound familiar?

Stimulating the thyroid artificially rather than finding out why it's not "feeling well" is akin to whipping a tired horse during the Kentucky Derby. At some point the horse is going to experience more pain, get angry, and may eventually even give up and stop running. The same can be said for the thyroid. If all we do to improve its function is to throw hormone-stimulating drugs at it, like levothyroxine, liothyronine, or desiccated thyroid extract, then the underlying causes will continue to wreak havoc on the rest of the body, and the thyroid will eventually wear out. To be sure, millions of prescriptions for these thyroid stimulants are written each and every year in the name of thyroid rebalancing. But is this really the answer to solving the thyroid malfunction puzzle? From this medical intuitive's perspective, absolutely *not*.

Forcing the thyroid to work harder by adding more thyroid-mimicking hormones may jolt the thyroid into action for a while but almost never address the true underlying causes of the thyroid misbehavior. So if thyroid stimulants are not the answer to bolstering poor thyroid function, how *do you* safely and effectively bring your thyroid back to health? The answer lies beyond the thyroid gland itself.

Most thyroid malfunctions are due to three commonly overlooked, yet profoundly important factors:

KEY THYROID DISRUPTORS

1. Unbalanced hormones
2. Low iodine levels
3. Revved-up immune system

Yes, it is that simple. When you identify and correct the three key thyroid disruptors, the thyroid will eventually balance itself without further assistance. If you feel the need for a more complex explanation than this or wish to be more thoroughly baffled than you already are, feel free to read some medical journals. If instead you want an easy-to-understand explanation of why your thyroid is not working properly, if you want the opportunity to live without prescription thyroid medications and still maintain your energy and weight balance, if you want to learn how to help improve your own thyroid health and your overall wellbeing, you've come to the right place.

We've already explored the critical importance of balancing the reproductive hormones and how low progesterone can have such a profound effect on thyroid miscues. Now let's take a closer look at how an angry immune system and low iodine stores play into some of the planet's most common thyroid misunderstandings, and your overall health and wellbeing.

Hashimoto's and Graves' Disease

Let's cut to the chase. The fact of the matter is that *hypo*thyroidism or low thyroid function, also referred to as Hashimoto's disease, and *hyper*thyroidism or high thyroid function, also referred to as Graves' disease, are autoimmune disorders; that is to say that these thyroid malfunctions are due to an exaggerated autoimmune response. What does that mean, "autoimmune response"?

The term autoimmune means that the body is actually fighting itself; it attacks itself in an attempt to protect itself from outside invaders. To put it more simply, when a foreign, unknown, or unwanted element, such as food borne or airborne foreign particles enter your body, your immune system will crank up to very high levels in a backward attempt to protect itself from harm. This potent and exaggerated immune response over time can have a deleterious effect on any of your internal organs, causing the tissue to become inflamed, and in the case of glands or organs, can even cause them to "burn out", in turn causing the gland or organ to stop working properly. In the case of Hashimoto's and Graves' disease, an angry and revved up immune system will attack and often destroy certain cells within the thyroid gland. The result is thyroid malfunction.

SIGNS AND SYMPTOMS OF HASHIMOTO'S DISEASE

- Weight gain
- Depression
- Mania
- Sensitivity to heat and cold
- Tingling of the extremities
- Panic attacks
- Heart racing, alternating with heart slowing
- Hypoglycemia
- Constipation
- Migraines
- Muscle weakness or cramps
- Memory loss

141

- Infertility
- Hair loss

SIGNS AND SYMPTOMS OF GRAVES' DISEASE

- Anxiety
- Eyeballs protruding
- Fatigue
- Frequent bowel movements
- Goiter
- Heat intolerance
- Increased appetite
- Insomnia
- Menstrual irregularities
- Increased sweating
- Nervousness
- Rapid or irregular heart beats
- Tremor
- Weight loss

These lists are not meant to be a comprehensive summary of all the symptoms that someone with Graves' and Hashimoto's may experience. There can be others.

WHAT'S IN *YOUR* GENETIC PROFILE?

Genetics play a key role in determining which glands or organs will be affected by an autoimmune uprising. With Graves' and Hashimoto's disease, the autoimmune response is targeted at the thyroid gland and typically reflects a genetic weakness in the thyroid, which is often carried down from your ancestors. In fact, it is not uncommon for individuals suffering from Graves' and Hashimoto's disease to have relatives who also suffered from these autoimmune maladies. Even if you're not certain about your genetic history, remember that a hundred years ago we didn't have names for these health conditions and yet many of them still existed, which means your ancestors may well have been afflicted but they didn't know what it was.

AN EQUAL OPPORTUNITY PREDATOR

Autoimmune uprisings are not picky, just specific. They don't just attack the thyroid tissues as in Graves' and Hashimoto's; the immune system can also attack any other gland or organ at the same time. It is not uncommon then to find someone with Graves' disease also suffering with rheumatoid arthritis or diabetes. While your angry immune system is revving up against your thyroid cells, it may also be taunting the cells in your colon. When this occurs, and it happens more often than most individuals realize, you may experience uncomfortable abdominal pain and discomfort from what they term "irritable bowel syndrome" or IBS, or Celiac, or Sprue, all of which are truly medical misnomers for an autoimmune response triggered by food allergies and other environmental stressors.

If you are so genetically inclined, you may also experience cellular stress from an autoimmune attack that affects the islets of the pancreas, which over time can create blood sugar imbalances called diabetes, a highly publicized and fear-generating pandemic that seems to be sweeping the planet. And that's just the beginning. The list of autoimmune-induced health conditions goes on and on. The fact is, literally every chronic health challenge and many acute health challenges have their root cause in autoimmune responses and the inflammatory process that goes along with it.

AUTOIMMUNE-INDUCED HEALTH CONDITIONS
(This is *not* a comprehensive list)

- CFIDS, Chronic Fatigue Immune Deficiency Syndrome
- Fibromyalgia
- Diabetes
- Rheumatoid arthritis
- Irritable bowel syndrome, a.k.a. Celiac, Sprue
- Sarcoidosis
- Guillain Barre
- Leukemia
- Polio
- Scleroderma
- Myasthenia Gravis
- ALS, Amyotrophic Lateral Sclerosis

- MS, Multiple Sclerosis
- Eczema
- **Hashimoto's disease**
- **Graves' disease**

YOU'RE NOT IMMUNE

The immune system is a powerful and crucial part of our defense system. Its job is to protect us from unwanted invaders and to maintain balance and harmony among all of the organs, tissues, and glands within each of us, and it does so faithfully and dutifully. But once this powerful organ system becomes over-stimulated from repeated exposure by undesirable and foreign objects, it can and will sabotage our very existence. In its attempt to protect us, our immune system will inadvertently ravage multiple organ systems unless and until you take proper care and precautions to avoid the autoimmune system triggers that can set it off. And they're all around you.

COMMONLY OVERLOOKED AUTOIMMUNE TRIGGERS

- Food ingredients and food allergies
- Heavy metal toxicity, including mercury toxicity from mercury amalgam removal
- Candidiasis, Candida yeast infection
- Viral infection
- EMF exposure
- Bacterial infection
- Any microbial infection
- Environmental toxicity from any source
- Chemical exposures
- Energy attachments in your home or workplace (a.k.a. ghosts)
- Lifestyle stressors
- Unhealthy relationships
- Prescription medications
- Genetics

WHO, ME?

Yes you. Each one of us at one time or another has been subjected to foods or other environmental toxins that have aggravated our immune system, even if you never realized it and even if you never experienced immediate overt symptoms.

Perhaps you had a headache after taking a prescription medicine, had muscle or joint aches after eating tomatoes, bell peppers, cheese, wheat or gluten products. Maybe you experienced heart palpitations or wheezing after eating at your favorite Chinese restaurant. Or you may have developed a rash, itching, or fatigue after painting a room in your house. These are all examples of autoimmune reactions, the body aggravating itself in response to interactions with unfamiliar or undesirable environmental toxins.

Sure, the traditional medical community may call these types of reactions a food allergy, a hypersensitivity reaction, or just a plain old fashioned "allergic reaction" rather than an autoimmune response where the body is actually attacking itself. The truth of the matter is that when your immune system has been subjected to repeated triggers from a foreign object, foods or toxins that it does not recognize, these can accumulate and culminate into an *auto*immune response that can lead to Hashimoto's disease, Graves' disease, or any other autoimmune condition imaginable.

YOUR FAVORITE CULPRITS

Some of us were lucky enough to be breast-fed as an infant. And being breast-fed during these important years was most certainly a boon to our tender immune system. Studies show that breast-fed children turn out to be overall healthier adults later in life. But there came a time in all of our lives when cow's milk became the mainstay of our milk intake, whether we were breast-fed or not. And as accustomed to cow's milk as we may have become and yummy as it may be with your favorite cookies, cow's milk and our immune system just do not mix. After all, we're not cows.

After decades of continuous exposure to cow's milk and other dairy products, the majority of the population in their 40's, 50's, and beyond, or the baby boomers, have developed immune intolerances to cow's milk. Millions of

145

individuals now experience digestive problems, including constipation, diarrhea, gas, pain, and bloating, or headaches, skin rashes, even mood issues from chronic exposure to this mega popular food allergen. And it's not just as simple as being lactose intolerant. In most cases, it's not the lactose our immune system rejects, it's the milk protein known as casein. And most immune systems are simply not happy about being subjected to this foreign milk protein.

And dairy is not the only familiar culprit. Allergies to wheat grain and gluten are a huge immune problem. Why? Because we've been exposed to it over such a long period of time and we continue to eat it daily in almost every food product we consume. Just read the food labels. It's everywhere, and in foods and beverages you would least suspect. A full 90 percent or the world's population is allergic to dairy and wheat and/or gluten, and most have no idea that they are. They also have no idea that these seemingly harmless food allergies are the root cause of many of the "mysterious" health symptoms they are experiencing. And we're not just talking about the well-documented physical symptoms of food allergies such as gastrointestinal problems like IBS, Sprue or Celiac, headaches, hypertension, or skin rashes. Food allergies are often behind mood swings, bipolar disorder, panic and anxiety, ADHD or Attention Deficit Hyperactivity Disorder, insomnia, and more. For a more in-depth look at how food and other environmental toxins are affecting your life, please read and explore my book "Extreme Clearing for Perfect Health".

Then there's the new generation of beings; those who were born in the late 80's, 90's and forward. In many cases this generation of souls is even more sensitive to environmental toxins, including foods and food additives, than even the baby boomers. A great percentage of these young individuals, referred to by some as indigo, crystal, and rainbow kids, suffer from severe dairy, wheat, and a multitude of other food allergies right out of the gate. Depression, anxiety, inability to focus, aggressive behaviors; this is just the beginning of their war with unhealthy foods and other environmental toxins that can ultimately lead to autoimmune wars, even starting at very young ages.

The bottom line is this:

- **Allergies to foods and beverages are the most common immune system disruptors on the planet.**

- **Immune disruption over time will lead to autoimmune problems at some point in your life.**
- **If you have genetic thyroid weakness, these autoimmune problems can lead to Graves' or Hashimoto's disease**

THE INSIDIOUS IMMUNE SYSTEM INVASION

In most cases these immune responses have been building slowly and escalating over periods of years, silently and insidiously, while you sleep and while you go about the daily affairs of your busy life. In fact it can take years, sometimes decades of exposure to these triggers to produce autoimmune responses, the level of which generate the cellular changes we call Graves' disease and Hashimoto's disease. But sometimes it can happen immediately. In some cases, the immune system can go haywire suddenly, unpredictably, and overnight, even decades after a single exposure to *any* autoimmune trigger and this is especially common in susceptible, ultra-sensitive individuals. And you are sensitive!

How quickly or how severely these autoimmune reactions present themselves will depend on your genetic wiring, your overall sensitivity as an individual on this planet.

JUDY, a short but spunky 58-year old woman of Italian heritage bopped into my office one day. A wise-cracking and lively lady, she reported that for over 10 years she had been wrestling with frequent panic attacks for no known cause, unpredictable and profuse sweating, heart racing, and difficulty sleeping. Her endocrinologist called it Graves' disease, and after one look at her eyeballs protruding abnormally from their sockets, I most definitely concurred.

Judy had tried several courses of the traditional therapies under the guidance of her endocrinologist, including the prescription medicines methimazole, propylthiouracil or PTU, and propranolol with little to no success. Edgy and a bit shaky, she seemed desperate to try anything, even alternative therapies to manage these disruptive symptoms.

After performing a thorough diet and environmental exposure history, it was clear that Judy had been exposed to numerous immune system triggers throughout her lifetime. Her diet was heavily laden with dairy and wheat products, plenty of helpings of fast food, and exposure to many other potential food allergens. Excited that we might be onto something, she confessed that she'd always had digestive problems, headaches, even skin reactions after eating certain foods for as long as she could remember, but she never made the connection to her thyroid symptoms, and neither did her other doctors. You could literally see the light going on in Judy's head. But there was more to Judy's autoimmune puzzle and the pieces were just starting to come together.

Suddenly she remembered that her thyroid symptoms seemed to get worse after she had remodeled her home a few years back. During that remodel period, Judy and the others in her home had been exposed to numerous toxic solvents used in the construction process. Within a week of the start of the construction her symptoms seemed to escalate rapidly with severe fatigue, heart racing, and unexplained sweating, and her headaches soon turned to migraines. This combination of food allergies and intense chemical exposures led to the autoimmune storm that took the cells of her thyroid by surprise, and to a full blown state of Graves' disease. Now it was time to clear the immune triggers and calm her revving immune system.

I started with a liver and gastrointestinal cleanse program to eliminate the toxic chemicals that had settled in her tissues. At the same time, I asked Judy to institute an elimination diet that included avoidance of all dairy, wheat, and tomatoes, all of which she was severely allergic to, and all of which she had been eating quite frequently.

We addressed her immediate symptoms with the natural medicine acetyl-L-carnitine to help moderate the uptake of thyroid hormone into her thyroid. I also added the B vitamin inositol to calm her nervous system, along with a potent digestive enzyme and probiotic to minimize the effects of any possible food allergy reactions and to tame her immune system. Iodine 400mcg daily was also added to feed and nourish her starving thyroid, as Judy's iodine levels had tested very low.

After adjusting her diet to include high protein and high iodine-containing foods, things began to noticeably change for the better. Within three weeks

time, Judy could not believe how much better she felt. No longer was she wired at bedtime; Judy soon began enjoying a comfortable eight hours of sleep nightly, something she hadn't experienced in over 20 years. Her excess sweating faded away, feelings of anxiousness and the panic attacks were no longer an issue and any semblance of headache pain all but disappeared. It took about four months to see everything return to a normal state but needless to say, Judy was more than pleased with the results.

I hadn't heard from Judy for several years until I happened to run into her at the grocery store just prior to going to press with this book. She looked vibrant and healthy and was elated to report that she was following my instructions to the tee and was still completely symptom-free. In fact, she was feeling so much better that she became a Harley Davidson groupie and was now cruising the country in full biker regalia with her new boyfriend, and enjoying every moment of it. Judy had beaten her "life sentence" diagnosis of Graves' disease simply by making the necessary immune-friendly changes. Her case remains a shining example of how to tame an out-of-control autoimmune disorder naturally.

HOW TO TREAT HASHIMOTO'S AND GRAVES' DISEASE (AND OTHER AUTOIMMUNE CONDITIONS)

If you have been diagnosed with Graves' disease, Hashimoto's disease, or any other autoimmune disorder, there is one key thing that you must accomplish to get yourself on the road to recovery:

Calm the immune system.

You can calm the immune system on your own, despite what the mainstream medical community might have you believe. And it starts by detecting and disarming the immune system triggers in your life right now.

Lest you forget, I have compiled a list of the key factors that need to be addressed when you begin your healing process with Graves' and Hashimoto's disease.

TIPS FOR DISARMING THE AUTOIMMUNE TRIGGERS

- Get food allergy-tested, then follow an allergy elimination diet
- Stay clear of electrical devices or any device that emits EMF or electromagnetic fields
- Avoid exposures to solvents, heavy metals, and other chemicals
- Reduce your life stress now
- Fix or clear unhealthy relationships, every one of them
- Balance your reproductive hormones
- Correct unhealthy diet habits
- Clear energy attachments from you and your living and work spaces; a.k.a. ghosts
- Clear all microbial infections immediately, especially Candidiasis
- Stay clear of all negativity in your life
- Begin a natural medicine immune balancing regimen under the guidance of your holistic practitioner

DISARM THE IMMUNE TRIGGERS

Once you've made the proper lifestyle modifications to disarm the immune triggers, it may take three to six months or more to achieve a full rebalance of your body's normal state. The actual length of time necessary depends on your genetic wiring and your current state of health. Please be patient. Remember that in most cases this immune system uproar developed over a period of years, even decades, and for some individuals, all of their years to date. So it may take a little time to see the response you're looking for, but it's definitely worth the effort. And don't hesitate to reach out to your local holistic practitioner to assist you in the toxin-clearing and immune-balancing process. They have the knowledge and the tools to help you get it done.

Need more help? Think you've already cleared *all* the toxins in your life, yet you're still not feeling better? Read my book "Extreme Clearing for Perfect Health". You will likely discover new ways to balance your health and balance your life naturally.

NATURAL TREATMENT METHODS

Please note that the regimens that follow are only the basic core regimens. The symptoms and underlying causes of Graves' disease and Hashimoto's disease can vary greatly among different individuals, hence the regimen will need to be tailored to meet the overall clinical picture and to clear specific immune disruptors. In many cases, natural antimicrobials or antibiotics and organ cleansers will be required.

Although self-treatment for these and other autoimmune miscues can be successful, due to the complexity of both of these conditions, self-treatment with natural remedies can be tricky and wrought with pitfalls, and is discouraged. Professional guidance is highly encouraged for optimum results, to minimize interactions and side effects, and to maximize results. Your holistic practitioner should be consulted to assist.

NATURAL MEDICINE TREATMENT REGIMEN FOR GRAVES' DISEASE

- **Inositol – lowers high testosterone, which can mediate a hyperthyroid state; nervous system tonic**
- **Acetyl-L-carnitine or L-carnitine – balances excessive thyroid hormone uptake**
- **Iodine- alleviates the low iodine state that can cause thyroid malfunction**
- **Melissa (lemon balm) – a natural sedative that calms the nervous system**
- **Fish oil – balances the immune system and reduces inflammation throughout**
- **B-Complex – strengthens and balances the nervous system**
- **Digestive enzymes – breaks down food products more completely to minimize immune responses**
- **Probiotics – balances the immune system and assists with proper food assimilation**

NATURAL MEDICINE TREATMENT REGIMEN FOR HASHIMOTO'S DISEASE

- **Progesterone cream - increases low progesterone levels to improve low thyroid function**
- **Iodine- alleviates the low iodine state that can cause thyroid malfunction**
- **Fish oil – balances the immune system and reduces inflammation throughout**
- **B-Complex – strengthens and balances the nervous system**
- **Digestive enzymes – breaks down food products more completely to minimize immune responses**
- **Probiotics – balances the immune system and assists with proper food assimilation**

THYROID BROKEN? FIX IT YOURSELF!

…with a little help from a qualified holistic professional. A diagnosis of Hashimoto's or Graves' disease from your local endocrinologist can be very disheartening and demoralizing to say the least. But that doesn't necessarily spell a life sentence of thyroid and metabolic misery. These common thyroid malfunctions can be balanced and reversed when the proper steps are taken. And it starts with you. Make a pact to change your diet. Make a plan to clean up the environmental toxins in your life, and do maintain a positive attitude about it all. And if you do choose to tackle these thyroid maladies without intervention from the traditional medical community, that doesn't mean you have to go at it all alone.

Schedule a visit with a qualified holistic practitioner of your choosing. But before you choose, make certain that your practitioner has a full and balanced understanding of the underlying causes of these two conditions. When properly detected and properly corrected, Hashimoto's and Graves' can simply become two names you'll never have to remember again.

HORMONE TRUTH:

The thyroid-targeted autoimmune disorders known as Graves' and Hashimoto's disease can be corrected by uncovering and correcting the underlying causes for the immune response.

The Iodine Enigma

Iodine? What does iodine have to do with hormone lies and thyroid misunderstandings? Well it may not sound like much, but the incidence of undetected iodine deficiency is one of healthcare's true enigmas. Why is that? That's because traditional medicine practitioners almost never consider low iodine as a culprit in thyroid malfunctions. That's unfortunate because in upward of 50 percent of individuals who present with thyroid malfunctions, low iodine levels are the primary culprit. And studies estimate that approximately 90 percent of Americans are iodine deficient. Sadly, most health care practitioners rarely address this prevalent nutritional deficiency.

So how does iodine fit into the thyroid malfunction picture? Iodine is an essential trace mineral that is required in the production of T3 or triiodothyronine and T4 or tetraiodothyronine, the two key hormones of this master gland. Because it's an essential mineral, iodine must be consumed on a regular basis in order to avoid a deficiency. When you become deficient in iodine, T3 and T4 can not be produced in optimum amounts and the thyroid can not work at its full potential, and this can result in *either* a hypothyroid or low state as in Hashimoto's disease, or a hyperthyroid or high, revved up state as in Graves' disease.

Low iodine levels are often the missing link in correcting most every thyroid disorder. In fact iodine is necessary to maintain many aspects of our health and vitality, including proper hormone balance, cellular health, mental sharpness, mood stability, immune health, and of course thyroid function. The truth is that iodine deficiency is responsible for over *50* different health imbalances, some of which may be plaguing you even as you read this. Here is just a partial list of health challenges and symptoms that can occur from an iodine deficiency:

SYMPTOMS OF IODINE DEFICIENCY

- Graves' disease
- Hashimoto's disease
- Immune deficiency
- Fibrocystic breasts

- Blood sugar changes including diabetes
- Fatigue
- Constipation
- Cancer
- Protrusion of the eyes
- Dry skin
- CFIDS, Chronic Fatigue Immune Deficiency Syndrome
- Fibromyalgia
- Low libido
- PCOS, Polycystic Ovary Syndrome
- Hair loss
- Foggy head, including confusion and memory impairment
- High cholesterol
- Menstrual upset
- Fear and apprehension
- Hot or cold sensitivity
- Brittle nails
- Skin reactions
- Anxiety
- Insomnia
- Depression
- Weight gain or weight loss
- **Goiter**

GOITERS

As you can see, the symptoms of iodine deficiency covers the gamut of health miscues, and likely you or somebody you know is dealing with an affliction because of it, and more than likely without realizing what's going on. And the more iodine deficient you are the more obvious and numerous can be the symptoms. And although some people may experience no overt symptoms at first, an iodine deficiency may still be brewing within and will eventually make itself known.

When iodine stores are too low, the thyroid will starve itself and in an attempt to correct the low level, in some cases creating a goiter, an overgrowth or lump of thyroid tissue that can protrude noticeably from the throat chakra.

Even upon examining their patients, many practitioners will completely overlook or ignore this unsightly and obvious goiter and fail to connect it with a simple iodine deficiency. And that's unfortunate because this missed opportunity has unnecessarily subjected millions of individuals, mostly women, to the throws of potent thyroid stimulant medicines such as levothyroxine and desiccated thyroid extract, in many cases for decades, when in fact all these individuals needed was about 10 cents a day worth of iodine supplementation.

And although it's the female gender that seems to make the most noise about thyroid malfunction, largely due to weight gain and fatigue symptoms, men are impacted equally by an iodine deficiency. It's true that in general women need more iodine than men in order to support breast health and other hormone-based imbalances; yet I would suggest that iodine deficiency in men is a huge health pandemic that has yet to reveal itself, largely because men are far less likely to report symptoms or even go to a doctor to discuss their health concerns. Men rarely discuss symptoms of depression with anyone, even their significant other; they rarely complain about anxiety, irritability, weight gain, and other symptoms, any of which may be the result of a simple and easily-correctable iodine deficiency.

WHY IS MY IODINE LEVEL LOW?

There are a number of reasons for low iodine levels, yet the primary cause is lack of dietary intake. The majority of the population is simply not consuming enough iodine in their diet. But there can be other reasons your iodine stores may be low, many that you may not have even considered. Perhaps you can identify with a few of them.

COMMON CAUSES OF IODINE DEFICIENCY

- Malabsorption syndrome
- Mercury fillings
- Fluoride supplementation
- Food ingredients
- Ultra-sensitivity
- Post-traumatic stress disorder (PTSD) from rape, war, violence, accidents

- Genetics
- Stressful lifestyle
- Environmental toxins, pesticides, heavy metals, chemical exposures
- Microbial infections
- **Poor dietary habits; iodine-deficient diet**

Wondering if low iodine levels are behind your thyroid malfunction? There are a couple of ways you can find out for sure. You could ask your traditional medicine practitioner to draw a blood sample to check your iodine levels, but that can be expensive and is often inconclusive. You could also employ the services of a qualified holistic practitioner to test your iodine stores using applied kinesiology. This method is generally quite accurate when performed at the hands of a skilled practitioner.

Then there's something you can do at home. It's called the iodine patch test. The iodine patch test is an excellent screening tool to determine if you or a loved one needs iodine supplementation. It's cheap, accurate, and non-invasive and it could be the ticket to improving your thyroid function and your overall wellbeing, and it can be performed in the privacy of your own home.

HOW TO PERFORM THE IODINE PATCH TEST

Likely there are those science-based clinicians out there who will call this test procedure a bunch of "fluff." I would suggest otherwise. Although this simple patch test will not provide a quantitative value as to *exactly* how low your iodine stores are, it will give you a good idea as to the severity of the deficiency, and that's what we're after. Once you've determined the approximate severity of the deficiency, you and your open-minded practitioner can better gauge the dose and duration of iodine supplementation that is required.

IODINE PATCH TEST PROCEDURE

1. Start by purchasing a bottle of tincture of iodine over the counter at your local drug store. Make sure it is *not* the clear iodine product but rather the dark colored iodine we all grew up with. You may have to ask the pharmacist since these products are often kept behind the counter these days.

2. Apply a two-inch by two-inch patch of iodine to the smooth skin of your inner arm. Allow this to dry completely without interruption. Avoid excess sweating or any clothing sleeves rubbing on this area. When you bathe or shower keep this area dry and free of any other substances such as soaps or shampoos.

3. Keep visual tabs on this spot at least once every hour to monitor how quickly the brown iodine patch is fading.

4. If the iodine patch disappears completely within eight hours or less, your body desperately needs iodine. If the spot completely disappears within 24 hours, you still need iodine supplementation, but in lower doses and a duration that can be determined by your practitioner.

5. In general, if after 24 hours the brown color has slowly faded but is still visible, medicinal supplementation of iodine is probably not necessary, but iodine supplementation through food stuffs is recommended.

EAT YOUR IODINE

A mild iodine deficiency can often be corrected simply by improving iodine intake through your diet. Unfortunately, the foods we consume are grown in soil that is depleted not only of iodine, but of many other minerals as well. Even so, there can still be enough of iodine in these foods to help put a spark back in your thyroid gland. If you are suffering from any thyroid malfunction, I encourage you to seek out and consume foods that are iodine-plentiful. You may be eating some of these already, but if you're not, take note of some of these healthy food options and make sure your diet plan includes them on a regular basis. If you believe you may be allergic to any of these foods, get food allergy-tested through applied kinesiology before you consume them.

FOODS HIGH IN IODINE

- Ocean fish, shellfish, clams, lobster, sardines
- Asparagus
- Carrots
- Tomatoes
- Rhubarb
- Potatoes
- Peas
- Mushrooms

- Kelp
- Lettuce
- Bananas
- Cabbage
- Egg yolk
- Onions
- Mozzarella cheese
- Garlic
- Sesame seeds
- Spinach
- Summer squash
- Swiss chard
- Turnip greens

When in doubt, just remember that sea greens contain some of the highest iodine concentrations of any food stuffs, and they offer other health benefits as well.

SALT OF THE EARTH

There is yet another method to help replenish and sustain healthy iodine levels. Use *iodized salt* when you prepare your foods and when you season your foods. That means that you will need to carefully read the labels on those round cardboard salt cartons to make certain that iodine has been added to the product. Please note that most grocery stores offer both varieties; salt that contains iodine, as well as salt that is iodine-free. If you want iodized salt, that is, salt that has been fortified with iodine, make certain the label clearly states that the salt is indeed iodized.

Although sea salt, or salt that has been harvested by evaporating sea water, does contain a small amount of iodine, it is typically an inadequate supply, and as with salts that have been derived from salt mines, iodine must be added to the compound to provide the necessary iodine nutrient. Hence non-iodized salt contains no iodine, and iodized salt has been fortified with potassium iodide or sodium iodide, or another iodine-containing compound. If you wish to boost your iodine levels, choose iodized salt when you use salt, with one caveat. If you have a severe and well-documented reaction to seafood, do *not* supplement with any form of iodine until you consult with a healthcare professional.

Iodine supplementation through food stuffs is most always a smart thing to do (unless you are allergic to iodine). However, sometimes it may not be enough to fully remedy your iodine deficiency.

I'M STUFFED

If you can't or won't eat high iodine-content foods, or if eating these foods on a regular basis still does not bring your iodine levels back to balance, iodine supplementation in the form of pills and liquids may be indicated. Iodine supplementation with medicinals, in addition to consuming iodine-containing foods, is often necessary if the deficiency has been in play for a long period of time, such as years to decades, or when treating the symptoms of Hashimoto's disease, Graves' disease, or if you have a goiter. In these instances, supplementation through food or the use of iodized salt alone is usually not enough to correct the condition.

TAKE A PILL

Supplementation of iodine using capsules or liquids is cheap, effective, and can work quite quickly when guided by the hand and mind of an astute holistic practitioner. In my practice, I routinely check iodine levels using applied kinesiology, and based on that finding will determine an appropriate dosage regimen.

The typical starting dose of iodine supplementation that I recommend is 150 to 200mcg (*micro*grams) of iodine daily taken on an empty stomach first thing in the morning. The dosage needed to improve symptoms will vary widely from individual to individual depending on several factors including overall clinical picture, any other health imbalances, age, weight, and genetics. Choosing the right iodine dose can truly be an art and a gift, and a healthy dose of medical intuition never hurts. Doses should be adjusted upward slowly and carefully and should be based on the measured iodine level, symptomatic improvement, and the potential for causing unwanted side effects in the individual.

Although iodine products are readily available over-the-counter on the shelves of health food stores, because of the potential for dosing miscues, I highly discourage dosing these products on your own. It is wise and practical to employ a practitioner who has experience in iodine supplementation. I say that with one caveat: There are some "holistic/integrative/alternative" practitioners who believe that more and fast are better. This is simply not the case, and this kind of thinking can actually be detrimental to your health. Before you employ the services of any practitioner, ask them to explain their methods for iodine supplementation and the dosing protocol they use. If they refuse to tell you or if they start with doses of more than 400mcg per day, it would be wise to seek out another practitioner.

AVOID AN OVERDOSE!

Although generally quite safe, there is a faction of holistic practitioners out there who believe in using mega-doses of iodine in their patients with iodine deficiency. What is a mega-dose of iodine? I have seen some patients come into my office taking doses of 25 to 50mg *(milli*grams) of iodine. These are enormous doses that in my opinion play no role in the correction of any level of deficiency. Although there may be certain studies that advocate these types of doses, and even companies who manufacture them, I find this practice to be out-of-bounds, inappropriate, and flat out dangerous.

A dose of 25mg is approximately 100 times the dosage level that I would recommend for a starting dose under any circumstances. It is not uncommon for individuals who use doses of that magnitude to experience panic and anxiety, insomnia, palpitations, chest pain, and other heart-related symptoms. When such an individual arrives in my office on such doses, I ask them to quickly taper off their iodine product. Then after approximately a week long break off all iodine, I will recheck their iodine levels and restart at no more than 400mcg daily. This type of conservative dosing will help prevent unhealthy over-stimulation of the heart and other organs and help ensure a smooth improvement in thyroid balance. In my experience starting low and working up slowly is the safest and most effective way to deal with any iodine deficiency.

FELICIA had been suffering from low energy and fatigue for years and was taking a moderate dose of levothyroxine, a prescription thyroid stimulant, for what her endocrinologist believed was a case of primary hypothyroidism. Yet despite 15 years of treatment with levothyroxine, Felicia's thyroid symptoms of fatigue and weight gain persisted. She decided to explore the natural medicine route.

While Felicia was recanting this unfortunate but all-too-common plight, I couldn't help but notice that she was sporting a prominent goiter, an enlarged area of her thyroid gland that was now protruding from her throat chakra. I also noted that Felicia was a bit clammy and quite fidgety. When I questioned her about the goiter, she explained that her endocrinologist never made mention of it, even though she complained time after time that she felt a lump in her throat when she swallowed. Instead her endocrinologist just kept bumping up the levothyroxine dose, year after year, until it could be bumped no further.

She confessed that due to her frustration with her endocrinologist's course of action, she recently engaged the services of a "holistic" medical doctor, and this new doctor had prescribed iodine to help improve her thyroid function. I was actually quite pleased to hear that someone was in the know about iodine supplementation, until I looked at her iodine bottle. The whole sordid picture became very clear. Felicia had been taking 37.5 *milligrams* of iodine every day for the past month, a massive dose that is well beyond what I recommend for any human. Before I could even utter my concern over the dosage, Felicia went on to tell me that she had recently begun experiencing frequent bouts of anxiety and new onset insomnia, after sleeping like a lamb for years. Then the dam broke. In tears, she confessed that she had gone to the emergency room just several days earlier for heart palpitations, skipped heart beats that she never had before. The emergency room doctor prescribed lorazepam, an addictive anti-anxiety medicine and sent her home, yet the palpitations and anxiety continued.

I reassured Felicia that these new symptoms were likely the result of mega dosing of iodine and instructed her to take no further doses. After a thorough check and review of Felicia's thyroid and iodine status, the verdict was in. Her iodine levels and thyroid function were way high, in fact, off the chart, as was her testosterone level, and had thrown Felicia into an artificially induced hyperthyroid state. Not only that, but Felicia's progesterone levels were very low.

As it turns out, Felicia had likely been suffering from very low progesterone levels since her full hysterectomy 15 years earlier. Ironically it was these low progesterone levels as a result of the hysterectomy that had been the originating cause of Felicia's fatigue, weight gain, and mood shifts. Unfortunately none of her healthcare practitioners ever picked up on that clue and instead a long term unnecessary course of levothyroxine was begun. The combination of an iodine deficiency from poor diet and genetics coupled with the lack of supplementation of the all-important progesterone cream after a hysterectomy, compounded by the long term use of levothyroxine, had all led to her cascading symptoms, and ultimately a goiter.

Felicia started on ½ teaspoonful dose of topical progesterone cream per my direction, plus a good size dose of inositol throughout the day to balance her high testosterone and relieve her feelings of anxiousness. After a five-day break from the mega doses of iodine, I started her on 400mcg of iodine to be taken first thing in the morning. I also recommended several supplement and dietary modifications to rebalance her metabolic and nutritional status. She happily complied.

It took about six weeks and several iodine dosage adjustments to get Felicia completely balanced, but that we did. Her goiter reduced in size to the point where it was almost undetectable and her energy levels increased dramatically over that period of time. Felicia called me several months later to inform me that she hadn't felt this emotionally balanced and energetic since age 17, and that was quite some time ago. To this date Felicia continues to do quite well and still takes an iodine supplement daily, the difference is that her maintenance dose is now 200mcg daily, and certainly *not* 37.5mg.

IODINE ALLERGY

There has been much to-do about allergies to iodine. So let's set the record straight. True iodine allergies are extremely rare. And the undue withholding of iodine supplementation either through food or dietary supplements can do you much more harm than your fear of being iodine-allergic.

Just because you believe you are allergic to iodine doesn't mean that you are. Many individuals have become concerned about iodine allergies after having a reaction when using intravenous contrast dye that contains iodine during a medical procedure, yet in most of these cases this reaction is due to the dye itself and not the iodine in it. Also, a good majority of individuals who experience reactions after eating shellfish are often just reacting to the proteins and pollutants in the shellfish rather than the iodine in these sea foods. Furthermore, those individuals who've had reactions to iodine supplements or certain thyroid supplements that contain iodine are often simply experiencing these adverse effects as a result of inappropriate iodine dosing, liver congestion, or adrenal fatigue.

That all said, if you believe you have a *true* allergy to iodine, it's important to discuss this fact with your practitioner before commencing any iodine supplementation with pills or liquid. On the other hand, do make certain that you do not unnecessarily deprive yourself from the health benefits of iodine supplementation just because you "think" you are allergic to iodine. Find out for sure. You deserve to feel better and live better. Iodine supplementation could be the elusive remedy to get you there.

HORMONE TRUTH:

Iodine deficiency is a commonly over-looked culprit behind many thyroid malfunctions, and iodine supplementation in the proper doses could turn your thyroid and your life around.

Goiters

Few situations are more perplexing to me than when an individual arrives in my office with a visible goiter. Most of these hapless individuals will tell you that their doctor never even remarked about the obvious protrusion in their neck and throat chakra. And from a medical intuitive and clinician's point of view that whole scenario is simply unacceptable and very hard to believe. How can you miss it?

Some patients will explain that their endocrinologists, specialists in their field, may have casually examined the thyroid protrusion, but in almost every case had nothing to say about it, and worse yet, *did* nothing about it. If you were lucky, they ordered a routine thyroid panel, which is most often inconclusive and useless in the diagnosis of a goiter. If you were *unlucky*, they ordered a biopsy; a painful, anxiety-laden procedure that often involves the use of a sharp needle, and that maneuver can inadvertently stimulate abnormal cell growth, something we want to avoid at all costs.

COMMONLY OVERLOOKED CAUSES OF GOITER

- Inability to express oneself
- Stifling relationships
- Environmental toxicity from any source
- Prescription thyroid stimulants
- Lifestyle stressors
- Mineral deficiencies
- Hashimoto's disease
- **Iodine deficiency**

WHAT IS IT?

The term "goiter" simply refers to the abnormal enlargement of the thyroid gland itself. Unfortunately when it comes time to diagnose and treat a goiter, the traditional medical community seems to make the whole process more complicated and convoluted than it needs to be. But managing a goiter doesn't have to be that complicated. Why? Because this overgrowth of thyroid tissue is almost always the result of one simple nutritional miscue:

A deficiency of iodine.

Yes, when it comes to detecting a goiter, it's often as simple as a careful visual inspection of the throat chakra, an inspection that should lead the astute practitioner to understand that iodine supplementation is most definitely warranted. Iodine deficiency is indeed one of the most commonly overlooked causes for a goiter, except for perhaps one other; failure to speak up.

EXPRESS YOURSELF

Because of the thyroid gland's proximity to the voice box, anything that causes an individual to suppress or squelch their feelings, emotions, *or words* can over time result in thyroid malfunction. In severe cases of squelching of your true expression, especially in sensitive individuals, this practice can lead to a goiter. This is especially true when the suppression has occurred either over long periods of time or if the suppression is related to a deep-seated or intense issue in your life. Not giving yourself permission to cry or not being allowed to cry, to laugh and to fully express other emotions due to fear of retribution or judgment is yet another form of suppression that can result in the formation of that unsightly goiter. This notion may seem a bit esoteric for some but I can assure that severe and longstanding suppression of your expressive nature can and will create negative cellular changes anywhere in the body, including the thyroid.

SAY IT AIN'T SO

If you suffer from a thyroid disorder of any kind, including the presentation of a goiter that either you or a practitioner notices, do whatever is necessary to restore your ability to speak up, and to express yourself in every way. That may require that you adjust the dynamics of one or more key relationships in your life. Or stated less tactfully, either work to fix the relationship in question or clear it from your life. Your health and happiness most certainly depend on it.

Sadly, despite all of the expensive high-tech medical gadgetry and costly blood and tissue sampling, all too many individuals with visibly detectable goiters will leave their practitioner's office with few answers, and even fewer results. And that is a travesty; because in many cases a goiter can be healed with about 10 cents worth of iodine daily.

ANASTASIA was referred to my office by a friend because of her longstanding and resistant weight issues. A pleasant, soft-spoken woman in her mid 50's, Anastasia was nearly in tears as we began talking about her decade-long plight with her burgeoning weight. Although certainly not obese by any standards, her inability to attain her desired physical stature had taken a great emotional toll on her self-esteem, and had even lead her to thoughts of "ending it all". That comment got my attention, and propelled me into a swift and thorough examination of her metabolic status.

As I began my routine visual scan of energy fields, I spotted something out of place in her throat chakra. There it was; a subtle, yet clearly obvious band of tissue around the lower segment of her neck. Even though she immediately dismissed this anomaly as fat around her neck, I could not agree. By my look, Anastasia was growing a goiter.

When I queried her further about this neck bulge, she confessed that she had pointed that area out to her primary care physician on several occasions, yet they were not at all impressed. To pacify her concern, they ordered a TSH (thyroid stimulating hormone) blood level, a blood test that is notoriously an inaccurate and useless predictor of true thyroid function. The TSH results indicated that Anastasia's thyroid function was just fine. *Just fine*? Clearly things were not just fine, and given Anastasia's deteriorating emotional and mental status, something needed to be done, and now.

Anastasia had been on a good size dose of topical progesterone cream for several years upon the advice of a friend, so her progesterone levels checked normal, yet balanced progesterone levels in this case were not enough to balance her waning thyroid function, and certainly not enough to deal with a buzzing goiter. But the mystery was solved once we discovered that her iodine levels were significantly low.

Anastasia started on an iodine supplementation regimen as I instructed, taking 225mcg of iodine once daily in the morning on an empty stomach. As often occurs during iodine replenishment, her body's requirements varied during the process, so close monitoring of iodine levels was indicated. In fact, it took several months of adjustments to her iodine supplement, *both up and down*, to get it just right. After four months of such adjustments, her iodine requirements stabilized and her maintenance dose of iodine remained at 450mcg daily.

Over that four-month period her goiter began to shrink and finally disappeared completely. I encouraged Anastasia to begin an exercise regimen of simple walking 45 minutes to an hour every day to help her tone and shed those pounds that were causing her so much emotional distress. And since her metabolic and nutritional status was now properly balanced from iodine supplementation, this simple regular exercise eventually got the job done. Anastasia was finally able to reach her goal shape and weight. To this day, Anastasia remains symptom-free and goiter-free and reports feeling more physically and emotionally balanced than she has in years. And you can too.

GOITER GONE

Goiters are unsightly, uncomfortable, and are a sure sign that something is amiss with your thyroid and metabolic function. Yet this overgrowth of normal thyroid tissue can be resolved and the gland reduced to a normal size using safe, gentle, and natural means. If you suffer from a goiter that has not responded to conventional treatment modalities, seek the guidance of a qualified holistic practitioner who is versed in the proper use of iodine supplementation.

HORMONE TRUTH:

Goiters are an obvious and sometimes unsightly reminder that your thyroid is not working properly, and that iodine levels and your ability to "speak up" may be compromised

Thyroid Stimulants: Levothyroxine, Desiccated Thyroid Extract, and Friends

If ever there was a class of prescription medications being used and over-used inappropriately, hands-down that would be the thyroid stimulants; levothyroxine and its cousin desiccated thyroid extract. That's because millions of doses of levothyroxine and desiccated thyroid extract are dispensed each year in an effort to jump-start a dragging thyroid gland, when in fact the thyroid gland is just fine and does not need to be stimulated at all. What does need to happen is to identify and balance the secondary or underlying culprits that are causing thyroid function to sputter. So why are the thyroid stimulant drugs so over-prescribed?

Simply, that's the way traditional medicine practitioners were taught to deal with symptoms of weight gain and fatigue, symptoms which are among the most common complaints women will have when they visit their doctor, especially menopausal and post-menopausal women. Unfortunately this practice of prescribing thyroid stimulants for weight gain, fatigue, and other thyroid-related complaints has become accepted as the standard of care and drilled into the minds of internal medicine, family practice, and endocrinologists across the globe.

Yet, this knee jerk instinct to immediately treat and stimulate the slacking thyroid has resulted in unnecessarily exposing millions of men and women to countless doses of a prescription drug they may not really need, and more importantly leaves the actual underlying causes of thyroid malfunction unattended. What *are* the primary underlying factors behind thyroid malfunction? Well, we've seen them before but let's review them once again, lest we forget:

THREE KEY FACTORS BEHIND THYROID MALFUNCTION

1. Hormone imbalances
2. Iodine deficiency
3. Revved-up immune system (autoimmune disorders)

SO HOW DID WE GET HERE FROM THERE?

Since its release in 1963, levothyroxine has been one of the most widely prescribed drugs on the planet with more than 70 million doses dispensed in 2011 alone. Levothyroxine is a thyroid stimulating hormone that contains T4, or tetraiodothyronine, one of the two key hormones produced by the thyroid. So it would make sense that if a woman reports having the classic symptoms of hypothyroidism, such as fatigue and weight gain, then a thyroid stimulating hormone should be prescribed, right? Wrong? What should be done instead is to supplement with topical or oral progesterone. That's because when progesterone levels are not at their optimum, T4, the inactivated thyroid hormone, can not effectively convert to the active thyroid hormone T3, triiodothyronine. It is this T3 hormone that will *naturally* jump-start the thyroid and remedy low thyroid symptoms, without the need for a direct and harsh thyroid stimulant prescription.

How big of a deal is this thyroid misunderstanding? *Big.* I would call it a world-wide pandemic, as evidenced by my findings where in over 90 percent of women who come to see me for weight gain and fatigue complaints, their measured progesterone levels were well below normal. And nearly every one of these individuals is either currently taking levothyroxine or has been on levothyroxine for those symptoms in the past.

MAKE THE SWITCH

Sounds pretty straight forward, doesn't it? Just ask your doctor to taper you off the levothyroxine or other prescription thyroid stimulants you may be taking and start yourself on topical progesterone cream to balance your progesterone levels. That would be ideal, but unfortunately this scenario rarely plays out in the world of traditional endocrinology. Instead, tens of millions of individuals worldwide continue to take levothyroxine or another thyroid stimulant to manage thyroid malfunction. And although taking a little pill every day may seem like a relatively harmless routine, because of the way the medical-prescription system works, it can be a very difficult vicious cycle to break.

The truth is, once you get on that dizzying medical carousel it becomes very difficult to get off it, unless you or your advocate speaks up and insists on it.

Among other reasons which we won't expound on here, the guilt and fear of challenging a "doctor's order" is a major factor that keeps this unhealthy cycle alive. Unfortunately, many individuals are afraid to question *anything* their doctor says, especially when these traditional practitioners insist that they must stay on these thyroid pills for life. I completely disagree with that line of thinking. Except for those rare cases where there is primary damage to the thyroid, or where the thyroid gland or a portion of it has been removed altogether, there is simply no good reason to implement a never-ending cycle of thyroid stimulant medicines without first addressing and correcting the underlying causes of thyroid malfunction.

FREE WILL

I honor the fact that we are a free-will planet; hence everyone gets to choose what they wish to do. If you choose to continue using levothyroxine and friends there are a few factors you need to keep in mind.

First, you will be required to take a pill every morning 365 days a year, and pay for them each month. Not everybody's favorite pastime.

Next, you will need to visit with your doctor every several months so that you can get stuck by a needle to monitor your thyroid function and you will pay for the privilege of doing so. They will likely determine your thyroid function using a blood test that measures TSH, or thyroid stimulating hormone, and you will pay for that privilege as well. The only problem is that the TSH test is at best an inaccurate and useless assessment of your true thyroid function and metabolic balance. This is evidenced by the fact that a large number of individuals with TSH levels within "normal" range *still* complain of many of their original and typical hypothyroid symptoms, such as low body temperature, weight gain, fatigue, dry skin, and others. Oh, the blood levels are quite healthy thank you, but the patient all too often is not.

If you were fortunate enough to employ the services of an astute practitioner, and you request it, they may agree to a blood test to measure T3 and T4 levels instead of or in combination with a TSH level. This is a more accurate way to assess your thyroid status, but unfortunately this is too rarely done in clinical practice, and therefore most levothyroxine dosage adjustments are decided from an irrelevant and often erroneous blood test result, the infamous TSH level. This practice often results in both *over*-dosing and *under*-dosing of levothyroxine, with some practitioners inadvertently pushing doses high enough to create a hyperthyroid state, without realizing what they have done.

And there you have it; the typical thyroid management protocol according to mainstream medicine.

SYMPTOMS OF THYROID STIMULANT OVERDOSAGE

- Sweating
- Insomnia
- Anxiety or panic
- Weight loss
- Palpitations
- Mood shifts
- Tremors
- Nausea
- Headache
- Hyperactivity
- Increased appetite
- Racing heart
- Hair loss
- Goiter
- Graves' disease
- Difficulty breathing
- Diarrhea
- **Osteoporosis**

GIVE IT SOME THOUGHT

Levothyroxine has been the mainstream treatment for low thyroid function for over 50 years, and although it may not be the ideal method to manage your thyroid misunderstandings, it does have a place in healthcare when used in the proper population of individuals. And please do be clear that your practitioner is not following this highly-engrained medical protocol of using thyroid stimulants to intentionally do you harm. Most of these practitioners genuinely and sincerely intend to do what's right. Then again, that is likely your intent as well. And you do have the choice to pursue other thyroid balancing treatment avenues. If you wish to break the thyroid stimulant cycle, you can. Reaching out to your holistic-minded medical doctor or qualified holistic practitioner is a good place to start. If, however, you choose to stay on your current course, there is yet another pitfall lurking out there, this one specific to the use of levothyroxine.

OSTEOPOROSIS

Like every other drug, levothyroxine is not without its share of side effects. One of the most common and insidious of these is low bone density, or osteoporosis.

Although it may not show up right away, eroding bone density is a fact of life for nearly everyone who takes levothyroxine for any period of time; hence it is not uncommon for women and men who take levothyroxine for long periods of time to have an increased potential for bone fractures, regardless of age. To remedy the occurrence of low bone density, traditional practitioners will often add yet another prescription drug to counteract the effects of the first drug, a practice that is all too common in the healthcare field. Alendronate, ibandronate, and risedronate are some of the commonly prescribed antidotes to combat falling bone density due to levothyroxine use, but these too are fraught with serious side effects of their own including documented increases in bone fractures in certain susceptible individuals. Now we've created an angry vicious cycle with no happy ending in sight. And you're certainly not alone in this predicament.

SUSAN had been taking levothyroxine 100mcg every day since the tender age of 18. At age 47 she appeared in my office complaining of exhaustion, fatigue, weight gain, and low mood. Like many women in this age range, Susan attributed these symptoms to menopause, yet she was still quite alarmed at the recent and rapid weight gain she was experiencing despite eating right and exercising daily. She had put on 45 unexplained pounds over the last two years, and that's what drove her to make an appointment with me.

Susan pointed out that her endocrinologist kept bumping up her levothyroxine dosage to counter the weight gain but that practice didn't seem to make any difference. Now on 175mcg of levothyroxine daily, Susan was also concerned about new symptoms that had recently sprung up, including increased sweating and feelings of apprehension, anxiety, and trouble falling asleep. She also made mention of increased bone pain following a recently fractured pinky finger. Like a yellow penalty flag at a professional football game, her story stopped me in my tracks. I sensed a foul had been committed and the player was levothyroxine.

I commenced a thorough check of Susan's hormone and thyroid status through kinesiology, and my suspicions were borne out. Susan's progesterone levels were very low and her estrogen levels were quite high. But the most damning evidence came from the results of Susan's thyroid status. Susan was in a hyperthyroid state, in this case, induced by the improper dosing of levothyroxine. Both Susan's T4 and T3 levels were high, in fact, off the charts, and by her report she was most obviously experiencing the effects of these elevated thyroid hormone levels.

After I reviewed my findings with Susan, she explained that her mother had experienced similar thyroid woes that persisted into adulthood, and she too had been on levothyroxine for years. As it turns out, Susan never really needed any direct thyroid stimulants at all, just a rebalancing of her genetically low progesterone levels which had been in play since age 18, and likely longer than that.

Puzzle solved, well almost. Because of Susan's recent bone fracture and her long-term history with levothyroxine, I felt the need to check her bone density. There it was as bright as day. Her bone density was as low as I could measure through my methods. She was a bit surprised to learn of this finding because her endocrinologist for whatever reason never recommended a bone density scan, and never mentioned that osteoporosis could be a side effect of levothyroxine. Nevertheless, these findings were enough to convince Susan to stop her levothyroxine after almost 30 years of being on it.

We initiated a taper of her levothyroxine medicine, but because Susan had been taking this medicine for such a long period of time it was imperative that we come off slowly and carefully in order to avoid rebound symptoms of low thyroid function. I explained to her that when the thyroid gland has been supplemented with thyroid hormones from an outside source for such a long period time, it literally forgets how to turn itself on, and this reboot can take weeks to months to fully complete. Yes, the process of weaning down the levothyroxine while weaning up her low progesterone took the better part of eight months. During this time, I suggested Susan increase her magnesium intake and supplement that with vitamin D 5000 units and vitamin K2 100mcg daily to help restore her bone density. We also agreed upon some important diet changes, including increasing her consumption of green leafy vegetables to improve her uptake of calcium, along with foods that were high in iodine, something her thyroid was starving for.

Over the first six weeks of this natural protocol, Susan's feeling of anxiety, insomnia, and the insidious bouts of sweating began to subside. As Susan's progesterone and estrogen levels came back to balance, so too did her thyroid function, without the need for any thyroid stimulants. As for her bone density, well that took a little bit longer to stabilize, closer to 18 months. But with a healthy diet, daily weight-bearing exercises, and a few natural supplements, we were able to bring her bone density into normal range.

Yet nothing brought more joy to Susan's life than the fact that finally, she was able to shed those unwanted pounds. Although she was losing only a pound a week, within a year's time she had completely lost the weight that didn't belong there.

IT'S OKAY TO BE DENSE

... at least when it comes to your bone structure. If you suffer from low bone density and you're taking or have been taking levothyroxine for greater than six months, you will need to decide which avenue of treatment you wish to pursue to deter the loss of bone density. Essentially you have two choices. You may slowly taper off levothyroxine over a three to six week period with professional guidance, or you may choose to continue taking levothyroxine as you have been. If you choose to remain on levothyroxine despite its bone-eroding potential, I highly encourage you to begin a bone density supporting regimen. I have outlined a basic one for you to consider:

BONE DENSITY SUPPORT REGIMEN

- **Vitamin D 2000 to 5000 units once daily with food**
- **Magnesium 300 to 1000mg daily in divided doses with food**
- **Calcium 500mg daily in divided doses with food**

- **Vitamin K2 100mcg once daily with food**
- **Regular weight-bearing exercises**
- **Plenty of green leafy vegetables for nutritional calcium**

A number of bone density formulas that contain a combination of natural bone building ingredients are also available and can be found at your local health food store or at your practitioner's office.

THE REBALANCING CRISIS

If you've made the decision to come off your thyroid stimulant medicine, there are a couple of rules you need to be aware of. First of all, do not stop taking these medicines suddenly. You must taper off of them slowly in order to avoid the symptoms of rebound hypothyroidism which can mean the return of the original symptoms such as fatigue, weight gain, dry skin, and other symptoms you had in the first place and likely with even greater intensity. Even during a slow and carefully planned taper protocol you may still experience some of this, although the symptoms are usually milder than with a cold turkey discontinuation.

This rebound syndrome can occur because it takes time for the thyroid gland to learn how to function on its own once again, without stimulant medicines. That's because the biology of the body moves more slowly than the pharmacology of the medicines. In other words, levothyroxine and any of it stimulant relatives will have left the body long before the thyroid processes the message that it needs to get back to work. This transitional period can last from several weeks to several months, even up to a year or longer, depending on your sensitivity and your metabolic wiring. Yet some individuals can begin to notice symptomatic improvement in thyroid function within a couple of *days* of initiation of the natural medicine regimen and the taper protocol. Either way, please be patient. Your body will find the correct setting on your thermostat if you give it the time and opportunity to do so.

For all of the above reasons and more, I encourage you to engage the services of a qualified and experienced practitioner to accomplish this process. They can help you understand, minimize, and manage the transitional symptoms that may occur with a thyroid stimulant taper.

DESICCATED THYROID EXTRACT AND FRIEND

Let's face it. Not everything works for everybody all the time. There can indeed be some individuals whose thyroid function will not fully balance even with the correction of hormone and iodine imbalances and modulation of the revving immune system, although I have found this to be a rare occurrence. If however all underlying aspects of thyroid malfunction have been properly addressed and the thyroid has not adequately responded, the addition of T3 hormone or triiodothyronine in the form of desiccated thyroid extract or liothyronine may be appropriate to restore normal thyroid function. That said, there are several issues that should be addressed with regard to the use of these two pharmaceutical agents.

First of all, both of these prescription medications can kick up thyroid function quickly and sometimes abruptly. This means that if the dose is too high or is increased too quickly you may experience symptoms of hyperthyroidism; namely heart racing, palpitations, insomnia, anxiety, sweating and more. As with all prescription and many natural medicines, it is recommended that therapy start low and slow. Please recall that not all people have the same dosage requirements, and that ultra-sensitive people like you must begin therapy with the thyroid stimulants and other medicines, slowly and carefully. That means use the lowest possible dose to gain the desired outcome and do allow enough time for a given dose to do its job. For most ultra-sensitive individuals, that will mean using doses that are ½ to ¼ the usual starting doses, or less. Be careful not to rush to bump up these doses, as pushing too hard and too fast can result in unwanted side effects. Also note that as with levothyroxine, blood sampling will be required to monitor T3 and T4 levels and to establish the status of thyroid function. Alternatively this assessment can be accomplished without blood tests using kinesiology conducted by your qualified holistic practitioner.

One last note regarding desiccated thyroid extract dosing; even though most practitioners have been taught to prescribe continuous daily dosing with these and other thyroid stimulants, it is my sense that short term or intermittent dosing can often be enough to jump start thyroid function. In some cases even a single dose or several doses properly spaced will do the job. Once the thyroid gland has been jump started, regular daily dosing *may not be necessary*. In either case, as with levothyroxine, these medicines should be taken once daily in the morning on empty stomach at least ½ hour before breakfast.

Secondly, it should also be recognized that just because the symptoms of low thyroid have been resolved with these medications, it does not necessarily mean that the stimulant therapy is appropriate, or that the underlying low progesterone, low iodine stores, or hyper immune state have been corrected. It simply means we have overridden these factors and forced, essentially "whipped" the thyroid into action. And this is not always the safest or healthiest way to accomplish metabolic balance. If your practitioner recommends desiccated thyroid extract or liothyronine for you, make certain that these three key underlying factors have been addressed and corrected first, and give your thyroid three to six months to respond to these adjustments. If after six months thyroid function is not substantially improved, treatment with these thyroid stimulants may be warranted.

THINK TWICE, MAYBE THREE TIMES

Thyroid stimulants may have a place in the world of thyroid rebalancing; especially desiccated thyroid extract, but their need and their use should be carefully weighed before initiating any therapy. Avoid the use of levothyroxine unless your practitioner has given you sound reason to use it for anything other than complete thyroid gland failure, or the absence of a thyroid gland. It is imperative to carefully and thoroughly correct the three key underlying causes of thyroid dysfunction; hormone imbalances, iodine deficiency, and a revving immune system, before initiating any thyroid stimulant regimen. This way you can avoid being caught in the web of hormone lies and the classic thyroid misunderstandings.

HORMONE TRUTH:

Thyroid stimulants are not the proper choice of therapy in the majority of individuals who complain of the symptoms of hypothyroidism. The underlying causes should always be addressed and corrected first.

10.

Breast Cancer Unplugged

When I set out to write this chapter of the book I wasn't exactly sure how I wanted to approach the topic. There is so much to say and so many ways to say it, and I wanted to remain "politically correct" in the process. So where do we start? How do we separate fact from fiction and the cure from cause? Most important, how do we open the door for optimism, courage, and confidence when faced with such a diagnosis, (I am intentionally avoiding the word "hope" since that word leaves the door open for possible failure) or even when faced with the *risk* of developing such a diagnosis because of family history?

Let's start with good news. Breast cancer is treatable when it's detected early enough, and there are simple and natural methods by which to accomplish this. There you have it.

The bad news, mainstream medicine has done little to educate the public about breast cancer prevention techniques except to sell mammograms. On the other hand, the medical community and its business partners have done a wonderful job of creating a "my-way or the highway" fear-based campaign that has driven literally millions of potential breast cancer victims running for cover, and racing to gobble up the only cure they sell: chemotherapy or surgery. But let's not go there.

We're not going to expound on the billions of dollars raised each year in the name of a breast cancer cure; yet none has been affected. We're not going to languish over the fact that pink ribbons are showing up in the most dubious of places, football player jerseys, beer cans, packages of diapers, cans of peaches, license plates, you name it. And so what if "cancer centers" are popping up like fast food restaurants in every major community in the country. It doesn't matter. What sales pitch you choose to partake in is a personal choice. What *does* matter is that you understand what you can do to keep breast cancer far away from you and the ones you love (which should be everybody). This is the breast cancer calamity unplugged.

HEAR YEA, HEAR YEA!

So how *do you* reduce your risk of inviting breast cancer into your life? From a hormonal standpoint, it boils down to two simple factors. If you want to reduce your risk for turning healthy breast tissue into abnormal cell growth, there are two key things you must do:

1. Reduce high circulating estrogen levels in your body
2. Reduce your exposure to estrogenic substances

This can be accomplished by taking an inventory of all the estrogenic triggers in your life right now, lurking around you without your knowledge or permission. That means staying clear of all hormonal prescription medicines, and washing your fruits and vegetables to remove pesticide residue that is often chemically similar to estrogen. That means not drinking or eating from plastic water bottles and other packages that contain estrogen-disruptive substances like the chemical byproduct BPA, bisphenol A. It means educating yourself about any and all of the estrogen-disruptors in your environment and avoiding them as if they were the plague, because at the end of the day it is a plague, a plague that is quietly and insidiously undermining your health and wellbeing.

But estrogenic over-stimulation is just part of the breast cancer picture, a picture that certainly no one wants to look at. So *don't look*. Instead take action. Take action by reducing the emotional and physical stress you've allowed into your life, by finally ridding yourself of all those stifled emotions you've held onto for years, even decades. Start by expressing yourself openly and honestly every day and all the time and speaking up when you have a beef with your romantic partner or your business partner, or anyone. Take action by making smarter and healthier food choices and by avoiding *all* unnecessary food additives.

Yet beyond all of that, there remains the simplest and one of the most important actions you can take. Start asking a lot of questions, especially of your healthcare practitioner; the tough questions like, why do I need to take prescription estrogen for my hot flashes or low libido or for my bone density, and why do I need a mammogram every year to two?

This line of questioning is sure to disrupt the status quo, and may make your practitioner feel a bit uncomfortable and even defensive, but it's necessary if you're serious about making a difference in your hormonal health. And once you've stirred up the status quo, and you will, you must also be willing to challenge the pat answers that are likely to follow. It means that one of the actions you take may include seeking out alternative thinkers and practitioners, those who focus on prevention and a holistic approach to breast health. And that's all good. Above all that, taking action means that you start paying attention to everything going on in your life; because many of those *things* could become a saboteur in your breast health. Besides, if you're not paying attention, who is?

COMMONLY OVERLOOKED CAUSES OF BREAST CANCER

- Prescription estrogen medications
- Lack of sexual expression
- Pesticides and food additives
- Environmental toxicity from any source, including tobacco smoke
- Hormonal birth control
- Over-nurturing others while under-nurturing self
- Emotional stifling
- Metal wired bras
- Poor nutritional habits
- Stressful lifestyle
- Hormonal imbalances
- Poor genetics
- **Mammograms**

START NOW AND STICK WITH IT

Start paying attention to the *real* breast cancer risk factors in your life right now, then start making new routines, develop healthier habits, and become aware, not of breast cancer but of breast *health*. There is a huge difference between the two, a difference that could save your life.

181

And it's never too late to start, because breast cancer does not occur overnight. In most cases it is a process that has been brewing or incubating over many years, and often over many decades. The window of opportunity in preventing breast cancer is always open, and I encourage you to take the opportunity to "look in" each and every day; especially if you have a family history of breast cancer.

But before you panic about the poor genetic history in your family, take a deep breath and relax. Despite what others might have you believe, you *can* overcome poor genetics. How? Make different and smarter choices than they did. Just because your sister, mother, aunt, or even grandmother experienced breast cancer in their lives does not mean that you have to. The truth is you can avert negative genetics by living smarter and healthier, and without fear. Fear is a powerful and potent emotion that can bring on any disease if unchecked, so don't let the fear of family history of hormonal cancers scare you into actually developing it. It's never too late to take healthy action now. Start by seeking out the services of a holistic practitioner to help you identify and correct your risk factors, including high circulating estrogen levels. Correcting high levels of estrogen alone can profoundly reduce your risk for developing those negative cell changes in your breasts.

SIZE MATTERS (AND NOT JUST FOR MEN)

Here's a topic sure to raise a few eyebrows, but none-the-less needs to be addressed. In general, women with larger natural breasts tend to have higher circulating estrogen levels than women with smaller size breasts. That's how the breasts became larger to begin with. Higher circulating estrogen tends to drive breast tissue growth and will ultimately manifest larger breasts. Higher estrogen levels also drive up the overall risk for developing negative cell changes in the breasts, including fibrocystic breasts and full blown breast cancer. This scenario is also prevalent in many post-menopausal women who, having emerged from their "change of life", now have a change in cup size, in this case, an *increase* in breast cup size. This is yet another example of estrogen dominance at play. I'm not suggesting that women with smaller breasts are not at risk for developing breast cancer. They most certainly can be, if all the triggers are properly lined up: poor genetics, environmental toxicity, stifled emotional angst, and more.

So why do some women grow larger breasts and other women not so much? Much has to do with family genetics; that is, if your mother, grandmothers, or aunts have larger breasts and have a history of cystic growth or breast cancer tendencies, then there is a good chance that you will too. Yet family genetics are just one piece of the breast cancer puzzle. Overall exposure to environmental toxins that mimic estrogen, often found in pesticides, food packaging and ingredients, and even in the environmental toxins that may have been more prevalent in the local environment that you grew up around, can drive up estrogen levels, and breast size accordingly, and thereby enhance your risk for developing negative cellular changes, up to and including breast cancer. Indeed, if you look at statistics for breast cancer rates by region, they are often tied to the incidence of toxic exposures from local industry, EMF exposure, and other sometimes unavoidable negative cell health triggers. Although it may not seem that way, it's no secret that breast cancer rates can and often do vary dramatically from region to region, town to town, and even from neighborhood to neighborhood, depending on the type of exposures in the immediate vicinity.

And although when faced with a young woman that has a strong familial history of breast cancer or fibroid cysts, traditional gynecologists will straight away order a mammogram, and often yearly follow-up mammograms, this may not be the healthiest course of action. Rather, I strongly urge you to consider more natural and holistic methods to detect and manage your risk for developing negative cell changes, many of which are outlined in this chapter and throughout this book. Unfortunately, instead, too many young women are needlessly subjected to the radiation and the disruptive proceedings of mammography, which is discussed below, and that can actually further increase your risk for developing unhealthy cell changes. In this medical intuitive's opinion, routine mammography screening for breast cancer starts at too early of an age, often starting with women in their early 20's, and is often performed too frequently. And as you'll learn, mammography may not be an appropriate breast cancer screening method for women of *any age*. There are better and safer ways to screen for and manage breast cancer prevention in high risk situations. If you or other females in your family have larger breasts and/or have a family history of breast cancer, or even breast cancer "scares", I encourage you to get your estrogen levels and the rest of your hormone profile carefully and thoroughly evaluated by a qualified holistic health care practitioner, even before you agree to your first mammogram exposure.

A CURE FOR BREAST CANCER?

Is there a cure for breast cancer? It depends on what you call a "cure". The traditional medical system will sell you its cure, and it's the same cure options in every situation, and they're not pretty: Cut it out, radiate it, and then infuse your body with toxic and expensive cell-killers to make sure it never comes back. At the end of the day the bigger question becomes, will you survive this type of 'cure"?

When your medical doctor recites those dreaded words, "you have breast cancer", they're going to offer you one line of defense and it goes like this: See your surgeon and see your oncologist. Is that all we've got? Is that all there is? From the perspective of this medical intuitive, the answer is absolutely *not*. Natural methods are available to help you both prevent and manage the cell changes associated with breast cancer, and these methods do not involve the use of toxic and expensive chemicals coursing through your veins.

PREVENTION AND MANAGEMENT TECHNIQUES YOU CAN LIVE WITH

Many holistic practitioners are armed with the skills and experience to assist you with a diagnosis of breast cancer, and these options most often do not include surgery or chemotherapy. Rather, they involve the use of potent vitamins and supplements, nutrition and lifestyle modification techniques, and yes, energetic, emotional and behavioral modification techniques that can affect real results.

Can the use of natural techniques actually stop and reverse abnormal cell growth? As with any other methods of treatment for any condition, every case is different, and depends on several factors: your family genetics, your current state of health and nutrition, and how soon the treatment methods are begun. It also has a lot to do with the willpower and the overall constitution and attitude of the individual afflicted. Those who maintain a positive and optimistic outlook tend to do better than those who are receiving treatment under fear or duress, which unfortunately is often the case. Many factors play into the success of treatment with breast cancer and other diseases as well, so choosing the perfect treatment plan is crucial and often a difficult, highly emotionally-charged process.

So how should you manage a breast cancer diagnosis? Choose the method that most resonates with you. However, while in deliberations, you will also want to weigh in the fact that some individuals are much more sensitive than others when it comes to the use of harsh medicines and treatments, and this factor alone may affect your rate of success. If this is you, remember that you do have options.

Please be clear, I am not presuming to lead you down one road or another when it comes to managing a diagnosis of breast cancer. You always have a choice. Some individuals will choose to partake in the traditional surgery and chemo combo *along with* holistic methods. Others go one way or the other. No matter which method you're leaning toward, I encourage you to explore all of your treatment options before you decide. One of those options should include a consultation with a qualified holistic practitioner. While you're there, do take the opportunity to discuss all your breast cancer prevention and detection opportunities. Doing so may help you avoid subjecting yourself to what is really the only breast cancer screening tool offered by traditional medicine, mammography. And although screening for breast cancer through mammography has become the mainstay in breast cancer detection, its safety and efficacy has been the subject of great debate in recent years, and for good reason.

THE MAMMOGRAPHY LIE

For decades now, the traditional medical establishment has suggested that mammography is the definitive screening tool in the fight against breast cancer, yet closer examination will reveal that mammography may not be the safe and effective screening tool that many in the healthcare field would like you to believe. The fact is that mammography exams are often inconclusive and inaccurate and have the potential to actually *increase* the risk of breast cancer. So before you jump onto the mammogram bandwagon as is so often recommended by traditional medicine practitioners, it would behoove you to take a closer look at the risks that are part of the package.

First, there is the issue of x-ray radiation exposure. Some practitioners and mammography proponents will suggest that radiation exposure from mammography is no more harmful than what one would encounter in a normal day strolling outside of your home. This is simply not true. Studies suggest that the exposure from a single mammography exam is approximately equivalent to *1000* dental or spinal x-rays. That is not a low dose exposure. And now even more recent studies reveal that radiation exposure from mammography increases the risk of developing *heart disease* in women who have no pre-existing risk for heart disease. And given the current practice of recommending mammograms every one to two years over the age of 40, that can add up to a mountain of radiation, especially since these exposures are cumulative over your lifetime. Do the math. How many mammograms have you already had in your lifetime? The truth is radiation exposure is a real danger and a serious limitation in the overall safety of mammography.

Then there's the issue of squeezing the breast tissue together to accommodate the procedure. This type of manipulation in and of itself can stimulate negative cellular changes that we wish to avoid. Anytime the breast tissue is manipulated in such a harsh fashion, especially when some tissue is already damaged and vulnerable as in the case of fibroid tissue in the breast, you increase the risk of setting off unregulated cell growth that could lead to full blown cancer, and we certainly don't need that. With all these risk factors finally surfacing with regard to the use of mammography in breast cancer detection, is the potential benefit even *worth* the very real risks?

AND THE ANSWER IS...?

Assuming you could justify the risk and see your way past the dangerous obstacles of radiation and breast compression, an even bigger and more important issue needs to be overcome. Is mammography even accurate? There is much well-founded concern that tumor detection using this method is often inconclusive and fraught with false negative and false positive reports. These types of miscues can leave the hapless and sensitive woman confused, frightened, and vulnerable, potentially resulting in the delay of treatment if needed, either natural or traditional.

At the core is the issue of whether or not mammograms can actually detect all potential abnormalities, and if detected, how to go about differentiating the findings. Or more succinctly, when it comes to finding an abnormality on a mammogram, the question becomes are we looking at fibrous breast tissue, usually the first thing to appear with high circulating estrogen levels, or are we looking at cancerous tissue?. Is it a life-threatening mass or just an innocuous and treatable fibroid cyst? Unfortunately, in too many instances the mammogram report leaves many questions unanswered and as a result often requires the frightened female to endure an even more fear-provoking procedure; the dreaded breast biopsy.

DIG IN

Aside from being painful and invasive, aside from creating intense fear within the individual, a breast biopsy or any biopsy poses a significant risk to the individual. What's the risk? Anytime we biopsy or agitate vulnerable and sensitive tissue or cells we run the risk of setting off unhealthy cell growth, especially in sensitive and susceptible individuals. Clearly this is something we want to avoid at all costs.

At the end of the day, many questions still remain unanswered with regard to the safety, effectiveness, and appropriateness of mammography. So, before you agree to throw yourself into the lion's den with a mammography exam, why not take matters into you own hands?

DIY- DO IT YOURSELF

You can and should be an active participate in your own breast health and the fight against breast cancer. Breast self-examination is a great way to start. These breast exams should be performed once monthly in the shower, in the privacy of your own home where you feel safe and comfortable. Although a procedure often recommended by gynecologists and other health practitioners, many women still fail to check their breasts in this fashion on any regular basis, and that could be a costly mistake. Simple monthly breast checks are at the forefront of early breast cancer prevention. It's easy to do and only takes a few minutes each month.

This self-check requires you to place your hand over your breasts in a specific manner so as not to miss any potential abnormal tissue growth. If you need help learning how to perform a breast self-exam, these procedures can be found on the internet or in a plethora of women's health books and magazines. And remember not to ignore any lump, bumps, or abnormalities you may discover during your self-exam. These should be immediately addressed with your gynecologist or holistic practitioner for further evaluation. Although most of these lumps and bumps are innocuous fibroid cysts resulting from high circulating estrogen, proper and prompt intervention can help prevent any further health repercussions and can assure early treatment of cysts or any other cell changes that may be lurking.

If, after completing your self-exam, you wish to get a second opinion about your breast health for any reason, or if you simply want some peace of mind, you can explore an alternative to the mammogram. It's a gentle and relatively inexpensive procedure that can be both accurate and safe, and poses none of the risks and pitfalls associated with mammography. It's called thermography.

BREAST THERMOGRAPHY

Although not yet embraced fully by the medical community at large, thermography is a far safer, non-invasive, and potentially more effective procedure than mammography in the detection of unhealthy cell changes. It's safer because thermography measures heat variations rather than using x-ray radiation to detect potential hot spots within the breasts.

The skilled thermography practitioner can visualize the heat variations using computer generated graphs to identify potential problems, not just within the breasts, but in other parts of the body as well. This method is safe, reliable, and relatively inexpensive, and in this author's opinion at least as effective in identifying abnormal breast tissue as a mammogram, perhaps even more effective. Thermography services are available in many larger communities throughout the country, and if you search the internet you will likely find a qualified thermography technician near your home town.

If you're looking for some clarity and confirmation about any breast discomfort you may be experiencing, consider employing the heat-detection method known as thermography. At the time of this writing, these services are still available without a prescription or doctor's order. So the next time your gynecologist tells you its time for your mammogram, tell them you'd prefer thermography instead.

EMILY seemed a bit spooked when I first met her in my office that day. An astute 52-year old professional, Emily had palpated several lumps in her right breast during a routine breast self-exam and was in a panic. Her discovery sent her running to her gynecologist's office and she had just come from there. By the look on her face, I knew something was up.

Her gynecologist immediately ordered a mammogram but Emily wasn't keen about the idea. Like many other women who are faced with a mammogram procedure, she was concerned about the radiation exposure, yet she was equally concerned about the bumps she felt in her breast and the possibility that they might be something other than fibroid cysts. Her concern was fueled by her family history of breast cancer, as her grandmother had died from the condition several years earlier.

After completing my initial evaluation with Emily, I did not sense that these growths were malignant, but given her family history and the fact that Emily's estrogen levels were running high, I wanted a more definitive evaluation in order to determine how to proceed. I suggested breast thermography. Although a bit skeptical at first, Emily agreed to give it a try. I reached out to an old colleague of mine, a gifted thermographer and a Doctor of Oriental Medicine and made the referral for her. Without delay, Emily started the natural estrogen balancing regimen I had designed for her which included DIM, topical progesterone cream, and calcium D glucarate.

She called me a week later after she received the results of her thermography exam. There was an obvious sense of relief and calm in her voice, and for good reason. The thermography exam had confirmed what I had felt so strongly. Emily's breast lumps were indeed the result of cystic growth driven by her high estrogen levels, and no malignancy had been detected. Ecstatic and relieved, Emily happily shared these results with her gynecologist who not only concurred, but was so impressed with the thermography process that she began employing it for many of her other patients.

Over our next few visits together, Emily and I discussed the causes of estrogen dominance, particularly the chronic over-nurturing of others while under-nurturing self. Emily confessed that she was guilty of this practice, especially with her children and she made a commitment to turn that around. And she did. Over the ensuing eight months, the combination of her estrogen balancing regimen and a new attitude toward her self and to life helped Emily finally achieve balanced estrogen levels. She was so inspired with these results and so impressed with the holistic approach we had taken with her condition, she embarked on a whole new career path in holistic medicine, so she could help others the way she had been helped.

When we last visited, Emily was building a private practice in natural medicine and couldn't be happier with her new career path. To date, her breast cysts remain undetectable. Thermography had saved the day and saved Emily from unnecessary radiation exposure and other potential health challenges. Thermography also provided us with the confirmation we needed to resolve her long-standing fibrocystic condition, and to keep Emily far, far away from the ravages of breast cancer.

DON'T OWN IT

Breast cancer is a negative buzz word that has infiltrated the very fabric of our modern society. And although the fear and trepidation of the mere mention of the term sends women everywhere into a cold sweat, or a *hot sweat*, it can be prevented and managed successfully using natural methods.

One of the most important things you can do to keep your breast cells healthy is to monitor and manage your estrogen levels with a qualified holistic practitioner. The next most important thing you can do is stay clear of all that "breast cancer awareness". Rather, seek to achieve breast *health* awareness instead. Give serious thought before you choose to partake or participate in any product, event, or activity that promotes highlights, accentuates, or otherwise brings to your conscious awareness this very negative disease label that has been dubbed "breast cancer". Why? Simply because whatever you bring into your consciousness you make part of your being, and breast cancer is most certainly something you can live without. Do your part to "unplug" the breast cancer fear machine. Make healthy and smart choices. They're out there.

Want to help keep breast cancer far from your life and the life of your loved ones? Stay clear of anything and anybody that brings the energy or even the thought of breast cancer into your energy field, and you will be healthier for it. Remember, when you label it, you own it. *Don't* own it.

WHAT YOU CAN DO TO PREVENT AND MANAGE BREAST CANCER

- Take calcium D glucarate 1000mg three times daily for 30 days, then 500mg twice daily until estrogen levels are within normal limits
- Take DIM, diindolylmethane, 100mg twice daily until estrogen levels are within normal limits
- Use progesterone cream applied topically at bedtime for 14 to 25 days as directed by your practitioner
- Take the vitamins and supplements recommended by your holistic practitioner to manage any cell changes that are already in progress. These may include IP6, vitamin C, maitake mushrooms, and others, and vary from case to case
- Reduce exposure to toxic environmental substances like plastic bottles that contain BPA, pesticides, and other chemicals and environmental toxins
- Avoid using *any and all* estrogen-containing products for any reason, including estrogen-containing birth control
- Experience sexual gratification and expression on a regular basis
- Consume plenty of cruciferous vegetables
- Avoid negative energies from negative people
- Avoid all negative situations and events
- Clean and wash all fruits and vegetables to remove residual pesticides and other toxins
- Speak up when you feel the need. Do not squelch your true feelings, emotions, or talents
- Avoid negative or stifling relationships, especially those with unbalanced sexual issues
- Do *not* over-nurture others while under-nurturing yourself. Treat yourself with respect
- Perform liver, colon, and other organ cleanses to clear heavy metals, pesticides, and other toxins
- Check and balance your hormones using progesterone and natural means only
- Minimize mammography exams and all x-ray exposures, including excessive dental x-rays

To learn more about how to clear *all* the toxins from your life, read my book "Extreme Clearing for Perfect Health".

HORMONE TRUTH:

Unchecked, high estrogen can eventually lead to breast cancer or other hormonal cancers in susceptible individuals. Even just a few weeks of exposure to estrogenic substances can be enough to trigger unhealthy cell changes in sensitive and susceptible women.

Mammography exams are performed too often, and in too young of a population, and are not a reliable method of breast cancer detection, often producing inconclusive or inaccurate results, while the process itself can increase your risk for developing breast cancer and other cancers.

11.

Sexual Expression and Your Hormones

Sex sells. This has been the credo of marketeers since the beginning of time. But did you know that sex also heals? Well it does. So if sex is not part of your life or you've decided to tuck it away in a shoebox for the past several decades, remember this: If you are not expressing your sexuality on a regular basis you could be making yourself sick. That notion follows one of my long standing theorems: When you suppress *anything* in your body for too long you create an opportunity for disease to set in. And you don't want that.

To be more specific, male or female, when you fail to express your sexuality for long periods of time you will eventually throw your hormonal, metabolic, and energetic systems off kilter, which can lead to physical, emotional, and mental disharmony. Not only are you setting yourself up for unpleasant health challenges down the road, you are depriving yourself of one of life's magical pleasures and spiritual treasures.

WHERE HAVE ALL THE FLOWERS GONE?

I have worked with thousands of hormonally-challenged individuals over the past three decades, and during that time, I stumbled across a very troubling trend among my female clients. More than 70 percent of them confessed that they had no sex life. Zero. Sex was simply an unimportant part of their life. Most troubling is that a good number of those who swore off sex were under the age of 40. Furthermore, at least half of all those who say they were going without, hadn't engaged in any sexual activity for long periods of time; five years, ten years, some even twenty years and longer. This whole dilemma took me by surprise, and I wanted to know what was behind it, so I asked them.

The mantra among all of these individuals was surprisingly almost identical regardless of their age, economic, social, or cultural status. And it went like this: Either they had no mate, had no social contact with a suitable partner, or chose not to engage in sexual activity for a host of what seemed to me as illogical reasons. In fact, most of these reasons seemed more like excuses to avoid the sexual encounter altogether, mostly out of fear from a variety of sources.

REASONS GIVEN FOR AVOIDING SEXUAL ENCOUNTERS

- Fear of being rejected
- Lack of self-esteem and confidence
- Feeling unworthy of experiencing pleasure
- Uncomfortable or embarrassed by their physical appearance or weight
- Fear of commitment
- Fear of transmittable diseases
- Too depressed to be interested in sex
- Male (or female) phobic due to past relationship traumas
- Too old for sex
- Too busy for sex
- Too tired for sex

And my favorite:

"It's been so long since I've had sex, I certainly don't need it now".

IT'S YOUR BUSINESS AND YOUR HEALTH

Some would argue that choosing to have sex or to *not* have sex is a personal choice and that it's none of my business, and they're right. I present this chapter not to insist that you become promiscuous or sexually inappropriate, but rather to demonstrate the magnitude of the "sexless" pandemic, and to drive home the point that avoiding sexual expression can be detrimental to your physical and emotional health.

And given the fact that nearly every one of my female clients is looking for answers to their hormonal miscues, this topic needed to be officially addressed. So let's address it. Lack of sexual activity can have a negative impact on your hormonal health. Want a solution? Revive your sex life.

So where have all the flowers gone? Gone to memories every one... so says the iconic song we all grew up with.

COMMONLY OVERLOOKED CAUSES OF LACK OF SEXUAL DESIRE

- Hormonal imbalances
- Thyroid imbalances
- Depression
- Fear
- Lack of self worth
- Prescription medicines
- Poor nutrition
- Hysterectomy
- Hormonal birth control
- Menopause
- Sexual abuse
- History of rape or other forms of PTSD
- Family or religious guilt
- **Chronic lack of sexual activity**

WHAT CAME FIRST?

The chicken or the egg? Did the stifling of sexual activity lead to all the hormone and organ imbalances, or did the hormone and organ imbalances lead to a lack of libido? The answer is YES! Both statements are true. It's a vicious cycle that can be both difficult to detect and difficult to break, unless and until you're serious about making changes in your lifestyle.

**Lack of sexual expression over time can lead to
low progesterone and testosterone levels and high estrogen levels**

And conversely:

**Low progesterone and testosterone levels and high estrogen levels
over time can lead to lack of libido, leading to lack of sexual expression**

Hormone imbalances from any cause, and we've covered them all throughout
this book, can and will lead to a lackluster libido, yet the opposite is also true.
Chronic lack of sexual expression can most certainly lead to hormonal
imbalances. And that paradox coupled with the myriad of other libido busters
in and around our life can propel anyone down a long and lonely path of
inadvertent celibacy. Why not break the cycle and enjoy all the attributes you
were born with?

ESTHER is a petite woman in her early 50's. She originally came to see me
to get some help with her irregular hormone cycles and the migraines that
resulted from her less than graceful arrival into menopause. Hers seemed like
an innocuous case of hormone malfunction, but little did I realize the
mysteries that would unfold.

After two years of working with her endocrinologist and gynecologist with no
success, they both discharged Esther, dubbing her dilemma a "medical
mystery". I saw it differently. Because each woman is uniquely wired with
very specific genetic coding, what works perfectly for one woman can quickly
fail to achieve any results in another. I felt that no one had yet found the right
combination of hormone modulators for Esther, but that was about to change.
Esther followed a very specific hormone balancing program I had developed
for her, that included topical progesterone cream, DIM, and several other
natural hormone modulators. Although it took almost a year of tweaking this
regimen, we finally did get it done. Esther's symptoms were finally under
control, except for *one*; one that she failed to mention altogether.

During one of our visits, she admitted rather casually that she hadn't had sex
with her mate in over 10 years. In fact, she'd had no sexual activity at all in
that period of time. When I asked her about this, she confessed that she loved
her man but had no interest in having sex with him. Sex was no longer
important to her. She was about to dismiss the whole issue when I explained
to her how lack of sexual expression often leads to the type of hormone
imbalances she came to see me about. With that, and a little friendly coaxing,
Esther agreed to explore the underlying cause of her sexual blocks while
under a light trance. Some call it hypnotherapy. I simply call it letting go.

While she was in this relaxed state I asked Esther to explore her true feelings about her relationship with her long-term roommate. The two weren't married, yet they had been together for over 20 years. Certainly many a happy couple has had successful long-term non-marital relationships, but something else was at play here, and we were both determined to find it. Finally after 30 minutes of gentle but poignant prodding, and in a profound tearful outburst, the truth revealed itself, as it always does one way or another. It turns out that Esther was dealing with her mate's long standing issues with alcoholism. For over 20 years, she battled *his* demons, spending all of her spare time and energy trying to keep him from killing himself with liquor. Even her precious weekend moments were consumed with "baby-sitting" him so that he would not injure himself on his weekend binges.

Despite wanting to enter him into AA on numerous occasions, he pleaded with her to let him go it alone. Time and time again she caved in to his requests and instead chose to be his "mother". In so doing, she took on and accepted his deep anguish and despair, the same anguish and despair that drove *him* to the bottle. Twenty-five years of this kind of emotional neglect had left Esther feeling passionless, emotionless, and in the end, sexless. Sex became the last thing on her mind for a variety of reasons, not the least of which is the fact that she felt like his caregiver and mother rather than a romantic partner.

It was painful but quick. Once Esther accepted this realization, a profound emotional block was released and things began to change quite rapidly. Esther defied his requests to leave him be and sought help from outside professionals for his addictive tendencies. Upon my recommendation, she started him on 5-HTP (5-hydroxytryptophan) to balance his low serotonin levels, which was responsible not only for his feelings of despair and anguish, but also for his myriad of addictive behaviors. Esther finally learned to remove herself from his emotional baggage and began to spend more time doing things that she loved.

Her partner ultimately quit his drinking tendencies but unfortunately the relationship was too far gone to salvage. The emotional connection at the romantic level was gone and the pair split. Esther finally moved on, and as with everything else in life, it happened for a reason, and for the best, although it sure didn't seem that way at first. With her emotional demons finally cleared and her hormone swings in check, Esther has regained her lust for life, and for love. Her sex drive had returned after a nearly 25-year hiatus, and she went on to rediscover the beauty, pleasure, and the treasure of intimacy.

ARE YOU READY TO REDISCOVER YOUR PASSION?

Correcting hormonal imbalances is not the only thing you can do to restore your sexual prowess. Other less-obvious challenges in your life right now may be responsible for your lack of sexual appetite. And many of these are easily remedied if and when you are ready. So why not rekindle the magic that lies within each of us. Feed your appetite. If you don't have one, start by addressing these commonly overlooked passion busters.

1. Fix or clear unhealthy romantic relationships

So many individuals remain in unhealthy, often non-sexual relationships, or unsatisfactory sexual and romantic relationships often for financial reasons, or just to avoid being alone, or for other reasons that often don't seem justified. If you are in such a relationship you clearly only have two choices: You can either fix the issues that are pulling you apart; this means working it out through honest and open communication, or you can clear it.

What do I mean by "clear it"? That means accept the fact that you've tried your hardest and done your best to salvage the relationship, and now it's time to clear it from your life. You deserve to experience joy and satisfaction in your romantic relationships, in *all* relationships. If you're not getting that from your relationship and you feel it's time to let go, don't hesitate to do that. Languishing in relationships that aren't working is not only painful, it's keeping you from experiencing the full expression of who you are as an individual, not just sexually, but physically, mentally, emotionally, and spiritually. And over time these types of empty and stifling relationships can lead to real-life health challenges you just as soon avoid, including diabetes, depression, hypertension, and hormonal imbalances.

If you feel you've done all you can in your relationship, work toward an amicable resolution. You'll not only be doing yourself a favor, you'll be doing the other person a favor too, even though they may not see it that way at first. Sure, breakups are painful and sometimes costly, but in the long run they are less costly than missing out on a full and satisfying life. In the long run, dissolution of unacceptable relationships can bring new life to all parties involved, and restore self-esteem and dignity in the process.

2. Take down the "stop sign"

You may not realize that you're actually doing this, yet I have seen it happen countless times over the years. Literally millions of men and women everywhere are holding up an energetic "stop sign", an energy signature, a vibe that other people pick up on, even when you're not consciously aware that you're doing it. This energy vibe is a signal from your aura, your personal energy field that's shouting out, "Don't look at me. I'm not available and I'm not interested".

If you're not satisfied with your current relationship, if you have no current relationship and are just angry and frustrated with yourself, your circumstances, or the rest of the world, you are sending out an energetic stop sign that others can easily sense, even when you do not. They don't know why they feel your stop sign vibe, but they do. And this negative energy keeps others from wanting to be with you, or even being around you. Is this the signal *you're* sending out? Is this the message you want others to get?

Start paying attention to the energetic message you're sending out when you're around others, especially when you are around someone that you wish to attract to you. Pay attention to your stop sign. When you're ready to accept another person into your life, when you're ready to engage and enjoy the pleasure of sexual commune with another at any level, and I encourage you to consider doing just that for your own health and wellbeing, then put up the "go" sign, the green light, the positive vibe that will alert others that you are ready to receive, that you are "open for business"; the business of building a healthy sexual relationship. Try it. It works

3. Be yourself. Find yourself

When it comes to your sexuality, your job is not to keep up with the Jones's. Your job is to be yourself; to be as sexually expressive as you feel you should be. No more. No less. And only you know what that is.

Let's face it, we were all raised with different morals, expectations, and views about sex and sexual expression, and each of us ultimately senses the need to hold true to those values. So don't spend all that time and energy attempting to live up to someone else's expectations, and by all means don't try to emulate anyone else's sexual preferences. That's their agenda. As long as you are not malicious in your behavior and do not intentionally harm anyone in the process, there is no wrong way to be expressive in this realm.

If you choose to avoid sexual contact with others for whatever reason, then take matters into your own hands. We weren't born with the tools to please ourselves for nothing. If your form of sexual gratifications involves only you, then be grateful for that opportunity. Self-gratification can be just right for anybody whenever needed, and is certainly preferable over no sexual expression at all. There's nothing wrong with pleasing ourselves. It's all perfectly normal.

And if in your sexual searching you discover that you've had your sexual gender choices confused all of this time, accept that too. For some, this discovery may take them by surprise, for others it's something they have known from early on but may have failed to accept or act upon. It's all good and it's all healthy. No shame, no guilt. At the end of the day, healthy sexual expression is simply that, healthy sexual expression. So start being yourself today. You may be surprised to discover a part of you that you didn't know existed; that passionate, sexual being that's been trapped inside of you all of these years. Maybe it's time to get reacquainted.

4. Get your hormones balanced

That's the big message of this book; we are only as happy as our hormones. But for many individuals, it's sometimes difficult to believe that something as simple as balancing your hormones can have such a tremendous impact on our sexuality. It can and it does. But when you really think about it, that's a big reason these hormones exist in the first place, to promote and manage our sexual expression. That's why I and others often refer to progesterone, estrogen, and testosterone as the reproductive hormones, or sex hormones. Keeping them in perfect harmony has everything to do with your sexuality.

If your sex drive has gone south for the winter, start your journey toward a healthy sex drive by getting your sex hormones balanced today. Break the cycle. Get your hormones checked and balanced by a qualified holistic practitioner.

BIOLOGICALLY NECESSARY

It's no secret that this planet is filled with many unique and different types of individuals with varied backgrounds, interests, skills, abilities, and belief systems. To that end, so unique and different can be our sexual appetite. Some individuals crave sex on a daily basis and even more frequently, others not so much. Still others are obsessed with sex, and must deal with these excesses in the same way as any other addictive behavior. Yet others have found a healthy balance in their sexual appetite.

Regardless of where you fit on the scale of sexual expression, no matter your level of sexual appetite, ravenous or "not right now, I have a headache", do remember this. Sexual expression is a necessary biological function that needs to be attended to on a regular and recurrent basis. Failure to do so can put your physical and emotional health in jeopardy.

Sexual expressiveness is an aspect of ourselves that should not be ignored, because as with many other things in life, when you ignore something long enough, it will eventually go away. Depending on circumstances, that can be a good thing or a bad thing. When it comes to your sexual expression, it can be an unhealthy thing. Remember, sexual expression is your birthright. Use it or lose it.

HORMONE TRUTH:

Lack of sexual expression over time can result in physical and emotional health challenges, including hormone imbalances, which can in turn create low libido and lack of sexual expression. It is a vicious cycle that can be diffused through natural means.

About the Author

Dr. Emil Faithe is a Medical Intuitive and Holistic Healer, and the co-founder of World Wellness Center in Albuquerque, New Mexico.

Dr. Faithe earned his Bachelor of Science degree in Biology from the University of California at Irvine in 1976, and went on to earn his Doctorate in Pharmacy from the University of Southern California in Los Angeles in 1981. Having practiced as a clinical pharmacist both in the hospital and ambulatory setting, Dr. Faithe always knew his pharmacy career was not going to be the standard fare. And he has most certainly not been disappointed. He began to explore the world of energy medicine, medical intuition, and natural medicines early in his career, setting the pace and the standard for the practical use of these alternative healing methods, while others in his field simply ignored their potential in managing the health and wellbeing of an individual.

During this period of time Dr. Faithe established a chain of professional health food stores in the Southwest, ultimately leading to the establishment of a private practice in holistic healing. This experience led him to his soul mate Susan, a powerful and gifted healer and intuitive in her own right. Together this powerful pair set out to change the course of holistic healing, and they continue to do so to this day, helping those who have not been helped anywhere else.

Using his well-rounded skills as a medicine man, both with pharmaceutical and natural medicines, Dr. Faithe has worked with nearly every health condition imaginable, and some that are not, helping thousands across the globe from all walks of life overcome their physical and emotional health challenges. Over the decades he has incorporated his gift of intuitive observation to help detect and resolve the "medical mysteries" of the world, in the process unraveling and unearthing the emotional and energetic causes of illness, and of wellness.

With over 30 years experience as a Medical Intuitive and Health Whisperer, Dr. Faithe works extensively with the ultra-sensitive individuals on the planet, helping them understand who they are and teaching them how to survive and thrive in the often challenging environment we call Planet Earth. He has been a keynote presenter at numerous health gatherings, and appears regularly on radio and television programs nationwide.

He is the author of the natural medicine primer "Natural Q's: A Guide To Healthy Living", a handbook for the consumer and for the health care professional just getting introduced to the field of holistic medicine; "Extreme Clearing for Perfect Health", a must-have guide on how to clear all the toxins in your life, especially those you never considered; and his most recent offering, "You Are Sensitive!", the unequivocal handbook and life guide tool for the ultra-sensitive individuals on the planet, individuals like you.

When not tending to the needs of the planetary inhabitants, Dr. Faithe enjoys working with the paranormal phenomenon, song writing, and playing DJ with the oldies music from the 60's and the 70's.

Dr. Faithe works with all health conditions and all ages, in person and long distance by telephone all across the globe. More information is available at his website: **www.truenw.com**.

CPSIA information can be obtained
at www.ICGtesting.com
Printed in the USA
BVHW082017291020
592032BV00004B/242

9 781626 463691